A Comprehensive Book on Experimental Pharmaceutics

A Comprehensive Book on Experimental Pharmaceutics

Mousumi Kar

Professor,
IPS Academy College of Pharmacy,
Indore, Madhya Pradesh.

Sujit Pillai

Professor and Principal,
GRY Institute of Pharmacy,
Borawan, Madhya Pradesh.

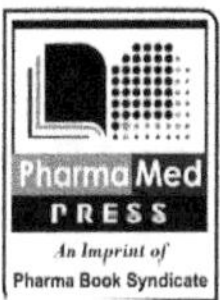

PharmaMed Press
An imprint of Pharma Book Syndicate
A unit of BSP Books Pvt. Ltd.
4-4-309/316, Giriraj Lane,
Sultan Bazar, Hyderabad - 500 095.

A Comprehensive Book on Experimental Pharmaceutics
by **Mousumi Kar and Sujit Pillai**

Published by

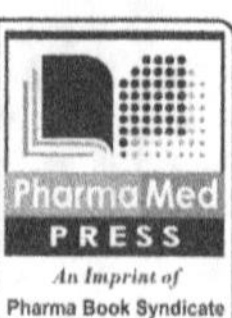

PharmaMed Press

An imprint of Pharma Book Syndicate

A unit of BSP Books Pvt. Ltd.

4-4-309/316, Giriraj Lane, Sultan Bazar, Hyderabad - 500 095.
Phone: 040-23445688, 23445600; Fax: 91+40-23445611
E-mail: info@pharmamedpress.com
www.pharmamedpress.com/pharmamedpress.net

ISBN: 978-93-88305-54-9

PREFACE

This book has been written keeping in view the undergraduate and post graduate students of pharmacy to provide a rapid reference towards experimentation and the use of ingredients for formulation. Nevertheless, it should be of value in most other cases where difficulties arise in the selection of excipients and during the analysis of the drug and formulated preparation.

For centuries, the drugs and excipients have been obtained from natural sources as inorganic minerals, plants and animals but their common name and general names have never been clear. This has been taken care in this book and a ready reference of commonly used excipients and their commercial available names have been mentioned.

Most of the universities that offer courses in pharmacy include introduction to the formulation science and analysis of drugs and dosage forms. Traditionally, a student knows about the formula but is usually not aware about the handling of equipments despite a change in the teaching approach.

This book will establish a ground work in pharmaceutical formulation of conventional and novel drug delivery systems, analysis of drugs and dosage forms and also in handling of equipments and instruments. An extensive coverage of practicals that are conducted along with inputs on technological aspects will make the material useful and appropriate for pharmacy students and researchers.

Mousumi Kar
Sujit Pillai

CONTENTS

Experiment – 46

Experiment – 47

Experiment – 48

Experiment 1

Hydrotropy Studies

A hydrotrope is a compound that solubilises hydrophobic compounds in aqueous solutions (by means other than micellar solubilization). The term *hydrotropy* was originally put forward by Carl Neuberg to describe the increase in the solubility of a solute by the addition of fairly high concentrations of alkali metal salts of various organic acids. However, the term has been used in the literature to designate non-micelle-forming substances, either liquids or solids, organic or inorganic, capable of solubilizing insoluble compounds. The chemical structure of the conventional Neuberg's hydrotropic salts (proto-type, sodium benzoate) consists generally of two essential parts, an anionic group and a hydrophobic aromatic ring or ring system. The anionic group is involved in bringing about high aqueous solubility, which is a prerequisite for a hydrotropic substance. The type of anion or metal ion appeared to have a minor effect on the phenomenon. Additives may either increase or decrease the solubility of a solute in a given solvent. These salts that increase solubility are said to 'salt in' the solute and those salts that decrease the solubility 'salt out' the solute. The effect of an additive depends very much on the influence it has on the structure of water or its ability to compete with the solvent water molecules. A convenient quantitation of the effect of a solute additive on the solubility of another solute may be obtained by the Setschetow equation:

$$\text{Log } \frac{S_o}{S} = K.Ca$$

where

S_o = solubility in the absence of additive

S = solubility in the presence of additive

C_a = concentration of additive

K = salting coefficient, which is a measure of the sensitivity of the activity coefficient of the solute towards the salt.

The study on solubility yields information about the structure and intermolecular forces of drugs. Use of the solubility characteristics in bioavailability, pharmacological action and solubility enhancement of various poorly soluble compounds is a challenging task for researchers and pharmaceutical scientists. Hydrotropy is one of the solubility enhancement techniques which enhance solubility to many folds with use of hydrotropes like sodium benzoate, sodium citrate, urea, niacinamide etc. and have many advantages like; it does not require chemical modification of hydrophobic drugs, use of organic solvents, or preparation of emulsion system etc. Solubility enhancement of various poorly soluble compounds is a challenging task for researchers and pharmaceutical scientists. The study on solubility yields information about the structure and intermolecular forces of drugs. Drug efficacy can be severely limited by poor aqueous solubility and some drugs also show side effects due to their poor solubility. There are many techniques which are used to enhance the aqueous solubility. The ability to increase aqueous solubility can thus be a valuable aid to increase efficiency and/or reduce side effects for certain drugs. This is true for parenterally, topically and orally administered solutions.

Object

Study of effect of solvent / cosolvent hydrotropic agents on solubility of given drug.

References

1. Maheshwari, RK., Solubilization of ibuprofen by mixed solvency approach, The Indian Pharmacist, 2009, vol VIII, No.87; 81-83.

2. Maheshwari RK, Chavada V, Sahoo K, and Varghese S., Novel application of hydrotropic solubilization in the spectrophotometric analysis of diclofenec sodium in solid dosage forms, Asian Journal of Pharmaceutics, 2006, vol I, Issue; 30-33.

Principle

Development of drug formulations for poorly soluble drugs is undoubtedly very important for producing patient-friendly formulations with high bioavailability. The bioavailability may be enhanced by increasing the solubility of the drug. There are different drug solubilization techniques. Such as, pH adjustment, micronization, micellar solubilization, co solvency and salting in, hydrotropy etc. Hydrotropes, co-solvents and water soluble solutes have been observed to enhance the aqueous solubility of poorly water soluble drugs. It has been demonstrated that synergistic effect can be obtained by mixed solvency concept. The use of hydrotropy can be utilized in titrimetric and spectrophotometric estimation of a large number of poorly water soluble drug substances. The mixed solvency approach discourages the use of organic solvents in large concentration (which may prove toxic) for development of a dosage form.

Requirements

Apparatus: UV Spectrophotometer, Beaker, Measuring cylinder, Volumetric flask & Stirrer.

Chemicals: Distilled water, Urea, PEG-400, PEG-6000, PEG-200 & PEG-4000.

Procedure

1. Accurately weigh 40 mg of Diclofenec sodium and transfer to 50 mL volumetric flask.
2. To this, add 40 mL of distilled water.
3. Shake the flask to dissolve the drug and make up the volume with distilled water.
4. Dilute the stock solution with distilled water to obtain various dilutions containing between 10-60 µg/mL.
5. Note absorbance at 276nm against reagent blanks to get the calibration curve.
6. Prepare blend (40%w/v constant) of solubilizers using varying concentrations of the solvents as shown below for Blends (1-4). Blend-1 containing urea, PEG400, PEG6000 and Sodium acetate, Blend- 2 contains urea, PEG4000, PEG200 and Sodium acetate, Blend -3 contains urea, PEG200, PEG400 and Sodium acetate and Blend- 4 contains urea, PEG400, PEG6000 and Sodium acetate.

Table 1 Blends and their Compositions

S. No.	Ingredients	% used in Blends			
		1	2	3	4
1	Urea	15	15	10	10
2	Sodium acetate	10	10	15	15
3	PEG 200	---	15	---	15
4	PEG 400	15	10	15	---
5	PEG 4000	---	---	10	---
6	PEG 6000	10	---	---	10

Observations

Table 2 Solubility of Drug in Purified Water.

S. No.	Concentration	Absorbance
1	10 ug/mL	
2	20 ug/mL	
3	30 ug/mL	
4	40 ug/mL	
5	50 ug/mL	

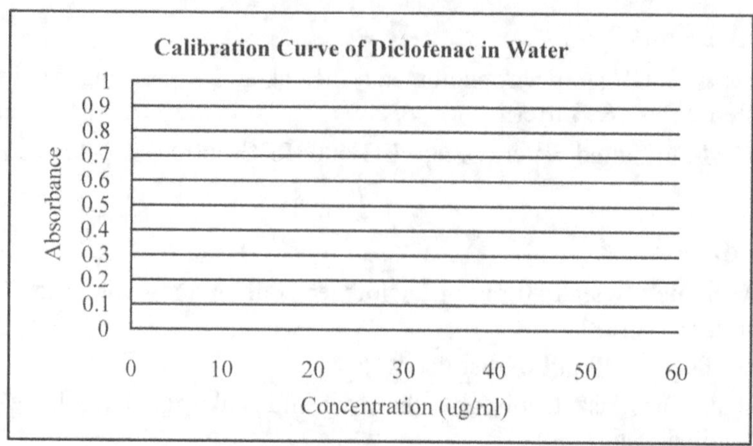

Fig. 1 Calibration curve of Diclofenac sodium in water.

Table 3 Solubility of Diclofenac Sodium in Different Blends.

S. No.	BLEND NO.	Absorbance	Saturated Solubility
1	BLEND NO. 1		
2	BLEND NO. 2		
3	BLEND NO. 3		
4	BLEND NO. 4		

Experiment 2

Drug Excipient Incompatibility Studies

Study of drug-excipient compatibility is an important phase in the pre-formulation stage of drug development. Drug-excipient compatibility studies represent an important phase in drug development. Before a drug substance is formulated into the desired dosage form, there is need for the formulation scientist to fully consider the chemical structure of the drug substance, the type of delivery system required and the proposed manufacturing process. Drug substances are usually combined with excipients which serve different and specialized purpose. Although excipients are pharmacologically inert, they can undergo chemical reactions and physical interactions with drug substances under favourable environmental conditions. These interactions can lead to instability resulting in the formation of new entities with different physicochemical properties and pharmacological effects.

Drug-excipient compatibility studies have been used as an approach for accepting/rejecting excipients for use in pharmaceutical formulations, thus allowing the rapid optimization of a dosage form with respect to patentability, processing, drug release, elegance, and physicochemical stability. In order to obtain rapid stability assessment of drug and excipients, drug stability, are investigated under the stress condition according to standard protocol and/or existing knowledge on potential degradation pathway or incompatibilities.

The potential interactions between drugs and excipients have effects on the chemical, physical, bioavailability and stability of the dosage form. Excipients are substances which are included along with the Active Pharmaceutical Ingredient (API) in dosage forms. Most excipients have no direct pharmacological action but are important for facilitating the administration, modulating the release of the active component and stabilizing API against degradation. However, inappropriate excipients can also give rise to inadvertent and/or unintended effects which can affect the chemical nature, the stability and the bioavailability of the API, and consequently, their therapeutic efficacy and safety. The incompatibility may be physical, chemical or therapeutic in nature.

Analytical Techniques Used to Detect Drug-Excipient Compatibility include:

Thermal methods of analyses: using Differential scanning calorimetry (DSC), Isothermal microcalorimetry or Hot stage microscopy (HSM)

Spectroscopic techniques: Vibrational spectroscopy as FT-IR Spectroscopy, Diffuse Reflectance Spectroscopy (DRS), Powder X-ray diffraction (PXRD) or Solid state nuclear magnetic resonance spectroscopy (ss NMR)

Microscopic technique: using Scanning electron microscopy (SEM)

Chromatography: using Self-Interactive Chromatography (SIC), Thin Layer Chromatography (TLC) or High-Performance Liquid Chromatography (HPLC).

Object: Study drug excipient compatibility of given drug with commonly used excipients

References

1. Indian Pharmacopoeia, Ministry of Health and Family Welfare, Ghaziabad, edition-VIII, 2014, Vol II, 1154.

2. Soni S., Drug excipient compatibility studies, CBS publisher, edition-I, 2012, Vol I; 201.

Requirement

TLC plates, Silica, Paracetamol sample. Different types of diluents, beaker, and pipette.

Drug: Paracetamol

Excipients: Starch, lactose and magnesium stearate

Mobile phase: 65% $CHCl_3$, 25% Acetone and 10% Toluene.

Apparatus

Flat glass plates of appropriate dimensions, an aligning tray, a spreader, a developing chamber, adsorbent, graduated micropipettes, a reagent sprayer, UV light source.

Theory

Study of drug - excipient compatibility is an important process in development stage of dosage forms. Incompatibility between drugs and excipients alter drug stability and bioavailability and there by affect their safety and efficacy. Dosage form is a pharmaceutical drug delivery system, which is a combination of drug(s) and non-drug components called as excipients. Thin layer chromatography is a technique in which a solute undergoes distribution between two phases, a stationary phase acting through adsorption and a mobile phase in the form of a liquid. The adsorbent is relatively thin and uniform layer of dry finely powdered material applied to a glass, plastic or metal sheet or plate. Glass plates are most commonly used. Separation may also be achieved on the basis of partition and adsorption depending on the particular type of support, its preparation and its use with different solvent. Identification can be achieved by observation of spots of identical R_f value and about equal magnitude obtained respectively with an unknown, a reference sample chromatography on the sample plate. A usual comparison of the size and intensity of spots usually serves for semi quantitative estimation. TLC techniques, now a days are important analytical tool for micro analytical separation and determination of the natural product.

Formula

R_f Value = Distance travelled by solute/distance travelled by solvent

Procedure

Preparation of TLC plate:

- Prepare 2% slurry of silica gel G
- Apply thin film of slurry to the TLC plate
- Keep TLC plate in hot air oven at 60°C

Mobile phase:

- Take Chloroform: Acetone: Toluene in the ratio of 65:25:10 and place in a TLC chamber

Saturation of chamber:

- Saturate chamber for 15 min

Sample preparation:

- Weigh accurately 1g of sample
- Dissolve it in 5 mL of ether
- Add 10 mL of ethanol

Method

- Apply small drop of sample to the TLC plate with the help of capillary
- Place TLC plate in TLC chamber
- Run mobile phase up to 3/4 distance
- Discharge plate and keep it in UV chamber
- Observe spot and mark it

Experiment 3

Solid Dispersions

The term solid dispersion refers to a group of solid products consisting of at least two different components, generally a hydrophilic matrix and a hydrophobic drug. The matrix can be either crystalline or amorphous. The drug can be dispersed molecularly, in amorphous particles (clusters) or in crystalline particles. Oral bioavailability of a drug depends on its solubility and/or dissolution rate, therefore efforts to increase dissolution of drugs with limited water solubility is often needed. Improvement in the dissolution rate of the poorly soluble drugs after oral administration is one of the most crucial challenges in modern pharmaceutics. Many methods are available to improve these characteristics including salt formation, micronization and addition of solvent or surface-active agents.

A solid dispersion is basically a drug–polymer two-component system in which the mechanism of drug dispersion is the key to understanding its behavior. In this review, we summarize our current understanding of solid dispersions both in the solid state and in dissolution emphasizing the fundamental aspects of this important technology.

Solid dispersion technology is the science of dispersing one or more active ingredients in an inert matrix in the solid stage to achieve an increased dissolution rate or sustained release of drug, altered solid state properties and improved stability. The solid dispersions may be-

Simple Eutectic Mixtures

Solid solutions which may be continuous, discontinuous, substitutional or interstitial in nature

- Glass solutions

- Compounds or complexes or

- Amorphous precipitates

The increase in drug dissolution rate from solid dispersion system can be attributed to a number of factors like particle size, crystalline or polymorphic forms and wettability of drug etc. One of the most important steps in the formulation and development of solid dispersion for various applications is selection of carrier. The properties of carrier have a major influence on dissolution characteristics of the drug. Solid dispersions may be prepared by various processes as fusion, solvent evaporation, fusion solvent method or super critical fluid method.

The advantages of solid dispersion include the rapid dissolution rates that result in increased bioavailability and a reduction in pre-systemic metabolism. Other advantages include transformation of the liquid form of the drug into a solid form. The disadvantages of solid dispersion are related mainly to stability issue, changes in crystallinity and a decrease in dissolution rate with aging.

Object

Prepare and evaluate solid dispersions of a poorly water soluble drug.

References

1. Chen S, Zhu J, Ma F, Fang Q, Li Y. Preparation and characterization of solid dispersions of dipyridamole with a carrier copolyvidonum Plasdone® S-630. Drug Dev Ind Pharm. 2007; 33:888–899.
2. Loftsson T, Vogensen SB, Desbos C, Jansook P. Carvedilol: solubilization and cyclodextrin complexation: a technical note. AAPS Pharm Sci Tech. 2008; 9:425–430.

Requirements

Chemicals: Drug, PVP K30, HPMC, Lactose, Microcrystalline cellulose, cyclodextrin etc.

Glassware etc.: Beaker, funnel, glass rod, measuring cylinder, mortar pestle etc.

Principle

Solid dispersion is one of these methods, which was most widely and successfully applied to improve the solubility, dissolution rates and consequently the bioavailability of poorly soluble drugs. The solid dispersion is based on the concept that the drug is dispersed in an inert water-soluble carrier at solid state. The solid dispersion has become an established solubilization technology for poorly water soluble drugs. Since a solid dispersion is basically a drug–polymer two-component system, the drug–polymer interaction is the determining factor in its design and performance. It is estimated that most compounds undergoing development at the present time are subjected to dissolution problems[1]. To meet this pharmaceutical challenge, various solubilization technologies have been developed including solid dispersions, nanocrystals, cyclodextrin complexes and lipid formulations. With accelerated increase in the number of FDA-approved products in recent years (Table 1), solid dispersion is now firmly established as a platform technology for the formulation of poorly-soluble drugs. Specifically, solid dispersion technology has been successfully applied to develop formulations with a high drug loading (*e.g.* 375 mg per tablet in Incivek) and/or containing drugs with a high tendency to crystallize.

Formula

S. No.	Name of Ingredients	Quantity Given	Quantity Taken
1	Drug	500 mg	
2	PVP	500 mg	
3	HPMC	500 mg	
4	Lactose	qs	
5	MCC	qs	

Procedure

A. Preparation of Physical Blend

1. Take drug and the polymer in the ratio of 1:1.
2. Sift through a 40-mesh (425µm) screen and mix together by trituration in a pestle-mortar.
3. Store in a desiccated environment.

B. Preparation of solid dispersions by solvent evaporation method

1. Take drug and polymer in ratio of 1:1, 1:3 and 1:5.
2. Dissolve the polymer in an adequate amount of methanol.
3. Evaporate the solvent rapidly by heating at temperature of NMT 50 °C, with surface airflow with constant vigorous stirring to form a uniform solid mass.
4. Crush the co-precipitate and desiccate under vacuum for 24 h, pulverize (again, after formation of a more fragile mass), vacuum desiccate again for a day.
5. Then sized into different sieve fractions and store in a desiccator, until use.

Evaluation

Drug content: Dissolve accurately weighed quantity of solid dispersions and mixtures of drug in 10 mL of methanol and stir on magnetic stirrer for 10 min. Filter the solution through membrane filter (0.45 µm), dilute suitably and analyze the drug content spectrophotometrically.

Particle size: Determine the particle size and particle size distribution of the samples using optical microscope fitted with microscope.

Dissolution Studies

The release rate of drug from solid dispersions can be determined using United States Pharmacopeia (USP) Dissolution Testing Apparatus 2 (paddle method). Take 900 mL of simulated gastric fluid maintained at 37 ± 0.5 °C and set 50 rpm. Perform the dissolution for 2 h. Take samples equivalent to a fixed weight of the drug for dissolution studies. Withdraw samples at regular intervals, filter through a membrane filter (pore size 0.45 μm). Replace with fresh medium maintained at the same temperature. Measure absorbance of these solutions spectrophotometrically. Determine the Dissolution Efficiency (DE) of the samples.

$$\text{Dissolution efficiency} = \frac{\int_0^t y\, dt}{y100\left(t_2 - t_1\right)} \times 100\%$$

Stability Studies

Carry out the accelerated stability study of prepared solid dispersion at 40°C/75% RH for a period of up to 3 months. Place accurately weighed amount of sample into glass vials with aluminum-lined caps and store in microprocessor controlled humidity chamber. Remove samples at regular intervals and evaluate for solubility, drug content, dissolution etc.

Film Coated Tablets

A film coating is a thin polymer-based coat applied to a solid dosage form such as a tablet. The thickness of such a coating is usually between 20-100 μm. It is possible to follow the dynamic curing effect on tablet coating structure by using non-destructive analytical methodologies. In pharmaceutical drug delivery of solid oral dosage forms film coatings are frequently applied. The motivation for coating dosage forms range from cosmetic considerations (colour, gloss), improving the stability (light protection, moisture and gas barrier) and making it easier to swallow the tablet. In addition, functional coatings can be used to modify the drug release behaviour from the dosage form. Depending on the polymers used it is possible either delay the release of the drug (such as in enteric coatings) or use the coating to sustain the release of the drug from the dosage form over extended periods of time. Film coating formulations usually contain the following components:

1. Polymer
2. Plasticizer
3. Colourant
4. Opacifier
5. Solvent
6. Vehicle

Functionality wise it is further divided into:

1. Immediate release coating
2. Sustained release or modified release coating
3. Enteric release coating

Tablet film coating technology conveys many benefits including improved packaging efficiency, prevention of cross contamination and reduced tablet breakage and chipping. And with a large variety of pigmented and non-pigmented tablet film coating systems available, coating may be done in a color of choice with a cost-effective coating that can also provide protection from light, moisture and environmental gases.

Tablet film coating is performed by two types, one is aqueous film coating (generally water is used as a solvent) and non aqueous film coating (generally organic solvent are used). Coating solution composition may affect the quality of final coated tablets. Optimization of composition of film coating solution is also required. This article discusses tablet coating process, film coating, process parameters, film coating advantages and applications, components of film coating, evaluation of film coated tablets, film defects etc.

The vast majority of the polymers used in film coating are either cellulose derivatives, as cellulose ethers, or acrylic polymers and copolymers. Occasionally high molecular weight polyethylene glycols, polyvinyl pyrrolidone, polyvinyl alcohol and waxy materials are also used.

Object

Formulation of film coated tablet.

References

1. Ratnaparakhi MP, Chaudhari S, Dhage K, Dhiwar SB and Bhore SS, Optimization of Coating Formula and Critical Process Parameter for Aqueous Film Coating of Tablet, International Journal of Research in Pharmaceutical and Biomedical Sciences, Vol. 3 (4), 2012, 1488-1496.
2. Roy A, Ghosh A and Datta S, Effects of plasticizers and surfactants on the film forming properties of hydroxypropyl methylcellulose for the coating of diclofenac sodium tablets, Saudi Pharmaceutical Journal (2009) 17, 233–241.

Requirements

Chemicals: Drug, sodium starch glycholate, microcrystalline cellulose, maize starch, PVP, colloidal silica, magnesium stearate, distilled water, hydroxyl propyl methyl cellulose, hydroxyl propyl cellulose, PEG 6000, Titanium di oxide etc.

Glassware etc.: Beaker, funnel, mortor pestle, test tube, glass rod, tripod stand etc.

Principle

The application of coatings to pharmaceutical solids has been practiced for over 150 years. Coating has been used in variety of pharmaceutical products such as tablets, beads, pellets, granules, capsules and drug crystals. It offers many benefits namely, improving aesthetic qualities of dosage forms, masking unpleasant odour or taste, easy ingestion, improving product stability and modifying release characteristics of the drug, for example, in enteric coating colonic delivery systems controlled release system and osmotic pump system. film-coating of tablets is a multivariate process, with many different factors, such as coating equipment, process conditions, composition of the core tablet, shape of tablets, coating liquid, etc., which affect the pharmaceutical quality of the final product. The side vented, perforated pan coater is the most commonly used coating device of tablets. So, process parameters greatly affecting the quality of final product as compared to the parameters related to pan coater. High quality aqueous film coating must be smooth, uniform and should adhere satisfactorily to the tablet surface and ensure chemical stability of a drug. Atomizing air pressure also affects the surface property of coated tablets. The spray rate is an important parameter which affects the moisture content of the formed film and subsequently, the quality and uniformity of the film. The inlet air temperature affects the drying efficiency (i.e. water evaporation) of the coating pan and the uniformity of coating. In the aqueous film coating process, tablets are exposed to wide temperature range and humidity variations that may promote undesired water penetration into the tablet core during coating or storage.

Formula

S. No.	Name of Ingredient	Quantity	Quantity Taken
	For tablet	Given (mg)	(mg)
1.	Drug	510	
2.	Sodium starch glycholate	12	
3.	Micro crystalline cellulose	07	
4.	Maize starch	10	
5.	PVP	30	
6.	Colloidal silica	07	
7.	Magnesium stearate	03	
8.	Purified water	qs	
	For coating		
1.	HPMC E5	08	
2.	PEG 6000	01	
3.	Titanium di oxide	03	
4.	Ferric oxide	0.5	
5.	Talc	qs	
6.	Purified water	qs	

Procedure

Preparation of tablet

1. Weigh each ingredient separately.
2. Transfer drug, SSG and MCC in a polyline container and mix well.

3. Add PVP in water and allow it to boil and then add maize starch to get slurry. Mix.
4. Pass the blend through sieve no 08 to get granules.
5. Dry the granules in a tray drier at 50°C for 15 min.
6. Pass through sieve no 18.
7. Add magnesium stearate and compress using a punching machine.

Preparation of coating solution

1. Transfer the required quantity of HPMC in a stainless-steel container. Add water and mix. For about 30 min.
2. Add PEG 6000 and stir for another 5 min.
3. Add titanium di oxide, talc and ferric oxide and mix for another 10 min.

Coating of Formulation

Transfer the prepared tablets to an R and D coater and coat with the prepared coating solution using the following condition parameter.

Spray rate- 8 mL/min

Weight gain- 2.5 to 3%

Preheating time- 10 min

Pan speed- 10-15 rpm

Air pressure- 0.6-1.8 Kg/cm^2

Air temperature- 40-50°C

Experiment 5

Effect of Surfactant on *In Vitro* Drug Release

In-vitro drug release testing, a measure of release of the active pharmaceutical ingredient (API) from the drug product matrix in controlled laboratory environment, is a key evaluation in drug development and quality control. It involves subjecting the dosage form to a set of conditions that will induce drug release and quantitating the amount of drug released under those conditions. In development, it is an essential test in assessing differences between prototypes, predicting the timeframe of API release, and modeling *in vivo* behavior. During this phase, *in vitro* conditions are generally selected to simulate *in vivo* conditions. In quality control it is used to assess conformance of a batch to pre-determined criteria at time of manufacture and to assess the long-term API release stability.

Surfactants are compounds that lower the surface tension between two liquids, between a gas and a liquid, or between a liquid and a solid. Surfactants may act as detergents, wetting agents, emulsifiers, foaming agents, and dispersants. The surface-active molecule must be partly hydrophilic (water-soluble) and partly lipophilic (soluble in lipids, or oils). It concentrates at the interfaces between bodies or droplets of water and those of oil, or lipids, to act as an emulsifying agent, or foaming agent. Other surfactants that are more lipophilic and less hydrophilic may be used as defoaming agents, or as demulsifiers. The properties of surfactants are such that they can alter the thermodynamic activity, solubility, diffusion, disintegration, and dissolution rate of a drug. Each of these parameters influences the rate and extent of drug absorption. Furthermore, surfactants can exert direct effects on biological membranes thus altering drug transport across the membrane. The overall effect of inclusion of a surfactant in a pharmaceutical formulation is complex and may be beyond those initially intended. The ability of surfactants to accelerate the *in vitro* dissolution of very slightly soluble drugs has been ascribed to wetting and/or micellar solubilization. The release of highly water-soluble medicinal compounds having fast rates of dissolution is of special interest.

Two possible mechanisms have been postulated as to why surfactants increase the rate of drug release from matrix formulations. Firstly, it is possible that the surfactant lowers the interfacial tension between the product and the dissolution fluid; secondly, it is possible that the surfactant acts as a wicking agent, causing the fluid to enter the dosage form; the surfactant may then dissolve and form pores (or other disruptions) from which the drug release may be affected. The magnitude of the increase or decrease of release rate remarkably depends on the type of surfactant and on concentration.

Object

Determine effect of surfactant on *in vitro* release of the given drug.

References

1. Park SH, Choi HK., The effects of surfactants on the dissolution profiles of poorly water-soluble acidic drugs. Int J Pharm. 2006 Sep 14; 321(1-2):35-41.
2. Applied Biopharmaceutics & Pharmacokinetics, Fifth Edition (Shargel, Applied Biopharmaceuticals & Pharmacokinetics) Leon Shargel, Susanna Wu-Pong and Andrew Yu.

Requirements

Chemicals: *Marketed ciprofloxacin tablet, SLS, Distilled water*

Glassware etc.: *Dissolution apparatus, Glass rod, beaker, Pipette*

Principle

Developing formulation using dissolution test methods for poorly water-soluble drug products has been an important task to formulation scientists. Problems encountered with poorly water-soluble drug products include a low extent of drug release and a slow release rate. General strategies to enhance their dissolution patterns rely upon either changing the dissolution medium pH or adding solubilizer such as surfactants and cyclodextrin derivatives into the dissolution medium. In rare cases, when the above attempts turn out to be unsuccessful, non-aqueous solvents are added into a dissolution medium. Despite having some health hazards, the use of surfactants in the tablet and capsule formulations for *in vitro* dissolution testing of water insoluble drugs has increased because of their mechanistic similarities to *in vivo* dissolution. Types of surfactants that are used in the dosage form to increase the dissolution include polysorbate 20/80, cetyltrimethylammonium bromide, sodium lauryl sulfate (SLS), lecithin, sodium cholate, sodium deoxycholate, sodium taurocholate, sodium oleate, and sodium glycocholate. Among these, SLS has been proven as the agent of choice because it is inexpensive, and it possesses good solubilizing capacity at relatively low concentrations.

SLS could enhance dissolution of poorly water-soluble compounds. The presence of surfactant influences the tablet disintegration rate, producing a finer dispersion of disintegrated particles with correspondingly larger surface area for drug dissolution.

An increase of SLS content increases the rate and extent of drug release. The increase of the amount of SLS gradually enhances the release of drug in dissolution study

Procedure

1. Preparation of 1 and 2% Surfactant Solutions

Take accurately weighed 100gm of SLS (sodium lauryl sulphate) and transfer into a clean and dried 100 mL volumetric flask. Add 20 ml of distilled water. Stir and make up the volume to 100mL. Repeat the procedure with 200 gm of SLS to get 2% surfactant solution. Label and keep aside.

2. Drug Release Study

1. Take 900 mL of dissolution media and maintain the temperature at $37° \pm 0.5°C$.

2. Add 20 mL of freshly prepared surfactant solution in the donor compartment of the experimental setup.

3. Now place the formulation to be examined in the surfactant media and carry out the dissolution process at 50 rpm.

4. Collect aliquots at regular time intervals and replace pre-warmed fresh buffer media.

5. Continue dissolution until plateau is achieved.

6. Analyze the drug content spectrophotometrically against reagent blank.

7. Repeat the procedure with 2% surfactant solution and also without any surfactant.

8. Plot graph taking time on X-axis and amount of drug released on y-axis

9. Compare the release profile to find out the effect of surfactant on the release rate of drug from the dosage form.

Table 1 Effect of 1% Surfactant Solution on Drug Release

S. No.	Time (min)	Absorbance (nm)	(Conc)	DF	Conc × 5 (mg)	Conc × 900 (mg)	CDR (mg)	% CDR
1								
2								
3								
4								
5								
6								
7								
8								
9								
10								

Table 2 Effect of 2% Surfactant Solution on Drug Release

S. No.	Time (min)	Absorbance (nm)	(Conc) µg/mL	DF	Conc × 5 (mg)	Conc × 900 (mg)	CDR (mg)	% CDR
1								
2								
3								
4								
5								
6								
7								
8								
9								
10								

Floating Tablet

Oral controlled release dosage forms have been developed over the past three decades due to their considerable therapeutic advantages such as ease of administration, patient compliance, and flexibility in formulation. However, this approach has several physiological difficulties such as inability to restrain and locate the controlled drug delivery system within the desired region of the Gastro Intestinal Tract (GIT) due to variable gastric emptying and motility. Gastroretentive dosage form can remain in the gastric region for several hours and hence significantly prolong the gastric residence time of drugs. Prolonged gastric retention improves bioavailability, reduces drug waste, and improves solubility of drugs that are less soluble in a high pH environment. The types of gastroretentive dosage forms are floating drug systems – effervescent and non-effervescent systems. Floating tablets prolong the gastric residence time of drugs, improve bioavailability, and facilitate local drug delivery to the stomach. Floating systems or hydro dynamically balanced systems are low-density systems that have sufficient buoyancy to float over the gastric contents and remain buoyant in the stomach without affecting the gastric emptying rate for a prolonged period of time and a better control of the fluctuations in plasma drug concentrations. Many buoyant systems have been developed based on granules, powders, capsules, tablets, laminated films and hallow micro spheres. Floating drug delivery systems are designed to prolong the study of the dosage form in the gastro intestinal tract and aid in enhancing the absorption. Such systems are best suited for drug having a better solubility in acidic environment and also having specific site of absorption in upper part of the small intestine. To remain in the stomach for a prolonged period of time the dosage form must have a bulk density of less than 1. It should stay in the stomach, maintain its structural integrity, and release drug constantly from the dosage form. The design of Floating Drug Delivery Systems (FDDS) should be primarily aimed to achieve more predictable and increased bioavailability. This ideal system should have advantage of single dose for the whole duration of treatment and it should deliver the active drug directly at the specific site.

Gastric emptying of dosage forms is an extremely variable process and ability to prolong and control the emptying time is a valuable asset for dosage forms. Several difficulties are faced in designing controlled release systems for better absorption and enhanced bioavailability. It is widely acknowledged that the extent of gastrointestinal tract drug absorption is related to contact time with the small intestinal mucosa. Thus, small intestinal transit time is an important parameter for drugs that are incompletely absorbed. Prolonged gastric retention improves bioavailability, reduces drug waste, and improves solubility for drugs that are less soluble in a high pH environment. It has applications also for local drug delivery to the stomach and proximal small intestines.

Object

Prepare and evaluate floating tablet for Ciprofloxacin

References

1. Desai S and Bolton S, "A floating controlled release system: *In-vitro in-vivo* evaluation" Pharma Res.1993; 10:1321-5.
2. Kar M and Reddy MS. Formulation and evaluation of floating drug delivery system for an antipsychotic Agent', PDA Journal of Pharmaceutical Science and Technology, 2006; 60(6): 389-94.

Requirements

Chemicals: Ciprofloxacin HCl pure drug, HPMC 100 cps, Gum Tragacanth, Ethyl Cellulose, Sodium alginate, Sodium Bi carbonate, Citric acid, Microcrystalline cellulose, Lactose, Magnesium Stearate, talc, Isopropyl alcohol.

Glassware: Beaker (250 mL), Measuring cylinder, Glass rod, Mortar Pestle, Volumetric flask (100 mL), Watch Glass

Others: Hot air oven, Disintegration test apparatus, Friabilator, hardness tester, Dissolution apparatus etc.

Principle

Floating tablets are retained in the stomach and are useful for drugs that are poorly soluble or unstable in intestinal fluids. The underlying principle is very simple. One attempts to make the dosage form less dense than the gastric fluids so that it can float on them by incorporating a number of low density fillers into the systems such as hydroxyl cellulose, lactates or microcrystalline cellulose. They also have an advantage over the conventional system as it can be used to overcome the adversities of gastric retention time as well as the gastric emptying time. These types of tablets are especially very useful in the treatment of the disorders related to the stomach. All those molecules with considerably short half-life can be administered in this manner to get an appreciable therapeutic activity.

Drugs that have poor bioavailability because of site-specific absorption from the upper part of the gastrointestinal tract are potential candidates to be formulated as floating drug delivery systems, thereby maximizing their absorption. The basic idea behind the development of such a system was to maintain a constant level of drug in the blood plasma inspire of the fact that the drug dose not underage disintegration. The drug usually keeps floating in the gastric fluid and slowly dissolves at a predetermined rate to release the drug from the dosage form and maintain constant drug levels in the blood. The concept of floating tablets is mainly based on the matrix type drug delivery system such that the drug remains embedded in the matrix which after coming in contact with the gastric fluid swells up and the slow erosion of the drug without disintegration of the tablet takes place. Sometimes for generating a floating system we even need to add some effervescent or gas generating agent which will also ultimately reduce the density of the system and serve the goal of achieving a floating system for onward drug delivery. These systems have a particular advantage that they can be retained in the stomach and assist in improving the oral sustained delivery of drugs that have an absorption window in a particular region of the G.I. tract. There systems help in continuously releasing the drug before it reaches the absorption window, thus ensuring optimal bioavailability.

Advantages

1. This type of drug delivery systems is especially very useful in the treatment of the disorders related to the stomach.

2. All those molecules with considerably short half-life can be administered in this manner to get an appreciable therapeutic activity.

3. This is a primary manner in which the bioavailability of a therapeutic agent can be enhanced. Especially all those drugs which get metabolized in the upper GIT.

4. It can be used to overcome the adversities of gastric retention time as well as the gastric emptying time.

5. The duration of treatment through a single dose, which releases the active ingredient over an extended period of time.

6. The active entity is delivered to the site of action, thus minimizing or eliminating the side effects.

Technologies based on Buoyancy Mechanism for FDDS

Non-Effervescent System

Commonly used excipients, here are gel-forming or highly swellable cellulose type hydrocolloids, polysaccharides and matrix forming polymers such as polycarbonate, polyacrylate, polymethacrylate and polystyrene.

One of the approaches to the formulation of such floating dosage forms involves intimate mixing of drug with a gel forming hydrocolloid which swells in contact with gastric fluid after oral administration and maintains a relative integrity of the shape and a bulk density of less than unity within the outer gelatinous barrier. The air entrapped by the swollen polymer confers buoyancy to these dosage forms. The gel structure acts as a reservoir for sustained drug release since the drug is slowly released by a controlled diffusion through the gelatinous barrier.

Effervescent System

These buoyant delivery systems are prepared with swellable polymers such as methocel or polysaccharides e.g. chitosan and effervescent component e.g. sodium bicarbonate citric or tartaric acid or matrices containing chambers of liquid that gasify at body temperature. The matrices are fabricated so that upon contact with gastric fluid, carbon dioxide is liberated by the acidity of gastric contents and is entrapped in the jellified hydrocolloid. This produces an upward motion of the dosage form and maintains its buoyancy. The carbon dioxide generating components may be intimately mixed within the tablet matrix to produce a single-layered tablet or a bi-layered tablet may be compressed which contains the gas generating mechanism in one hydrocolloid containing layer and the drug in the other layer formulated for the SR effect.

The floating dosage forms are kept in the stomach for extended periods of time the therapeutic agents are not immediately released after ingestion. Controlled release of such therapeutic agents from the dosage forms prevents enzyme saturation thereby improving the bioavailability of such therapeutic agents. So, it improves the bioavailability of by administering such therapeutic agent in a floating dosage from.

Procedure

Formulation

Formula

S. No.	Ingredients	Quantity given (mg)	Quantity taken (mg)
1	Drug	100 mg	
2	HPMC 100 cps	100 mg	
3	Gum Tragancanth	70 mg	
4	Ethyl Cellulose (25 cps)	25 mg	
5	Sodium Alginate	50 mg	
6	Sodium bicarbonate	60 mg	
7	Citric acid	40 mg	

Table *contd...*

S. No.	Ingredients	Quantity given (mg)	Quantity taken (mg)
8	Microcrystalline Cellulose	20 mg	
9	Lactose qs	500 mg	
10	Magnesium Stearate	qs	
11	Talc	qs	
12	Isopropyl Alcohol	qs	

Procedure

1. Weigh all the ingredients separately and keep aside.
2. Take a clean and dried mortar and add in ascending order of weight, the drug, polymers, gas generating agents and diluents.
3. Triturate thoroughly to get a homogeneous mixture.
4. Granulate by drop wise addition of isopropyl alcohol to get a soft dough.
5. Pass through sieves and collect the granules retained on Sieve No 22 and fines. Discard the percentage retained on Sieve No 16.
6. Dry the granules in preheated oven at 40°C and weigh them.
7. Add 5% of the fines to the granules and also the required amount of talc and magnesium stearate.
8. Mix thoroughly and weigh again.
9. Punch to get 500 mg tablets.
10. Store in an amber colored bottle in desiccator until use.

Evaluation

Precompression Parameters

1. % Yield
2. % fines
3. Angle of repose
4. Size of granules
5. Shape of granules
6. Colour of granules
7. Tapped density
8. Bulk density
9. Compressibility index
10. Hausner ratio
11. Post compression parameters:
12. Diameter of tablet

13. Weight and weight variation of tablet

14. Thickness

15. Drug content

16. Friability

17. Floating lag time

18. Floating duration

19. Dissolution time

Table 1 Pre-compression Parameters

Formulation	% Yield	% Fines	Angle of repose	Shape	Color	Size of granules
1						
2						
3						

Table 2 Post-compression Parameters of Tablets

Formulation	Diameter	Weight variation	Thickness (cm)	Drug content (mg)	Friability	Floating lag time (min)	Floating duration (min)
1							
2							
3							

Table 3 Dissolution Data

S. No.	Time in min	Absorbance	Concentration (X) µg/mL	(X × 5) µg/mL	(X × 900) µg/mL	Cumulative amount of drug released mg
0	0					
1	30					
2	60					
3	90					
4	120					
5	150					
6	180					

Experiment 7

Comparison of Antacid Activity

An antacid is a substance which neutralizes stomach acidity and is used to relieve heartburn, indigestion or an upset stomach. Antacids are available over the counter and are taken by mouth to quickly relieve occasional heartburn, the major symptom of gastroesophageal reflux disease and also indigestion. Treatment with antacids alone is symptomatic and only justified for minor symptoms. Antacids are distinct from acid-reducing drugs like H_2-receptor antagonists or proton pump inhibitors and they do not kill the bacteria *Helicobacter pylori*, which causes most ulcers. This medication is used to treat the symptoms of too much stomach acid such as stomach upset, heartburn, and acid indigestion. It is also used to relieve symptoms of extra gas such as belching, bloating, and feelings of pressure/discomfort in the stomach/gut. Simethicone helps break up gas bubbles in the gut. Aluminium and magnesium antacids work quickly to lower the acid in the stomach. Liquid antacids usually work faster/better than tablets or capsules.

This medication works only on existing acid in the stomach. It does not prevent acid production. It may be used alone or with other medications that lower acid production (e.g., H2 blockers such as cimetidine/ranitidine and proton pump inhibitors such as omeprazole).

Antacids usually come as a liquid, chewable gummy or tablet, or tablet that you dissolve in water to drink. They can be used to treat symptoms of excess stomach acid, such as:

1. acid reflux, which can include regurgitation, bitter taste, persistent dry cough, pain when you lie down, and trouble swallowing

2. heartburn, which is a burning sensation in your chest or throat caused by acid reflux

3. indigestion, which is pain in your upper gut that can feel like gas or bloating

Versions with magnesium may cause diarrhea, and brands with calcium or aluminium may cause constipation and rarely, long-term use may cause kidney stones. Long-term use of versions with aluminium may increase the risk for getting osteoporosis. When excessive amounts of acids are produced in the stomach the natural mucous barrier that protects the lining of the stomach can damage the esophagus in people with acid reflux. Antacids contain alkaline ions that chemically neutralize stomach gastric acid, reducing damage and relieving pain. Antacids may be formulated with other active ingredients such as simethi cone to control gas or alginic acid to act as a physical barrier to acid.

Antacids are typically safe for most people. But in cases as, people with heart failure may have sodium restrictions to help decrease fluid build-up. These antacids often contain a lot of sodium, though. These people should ask their doctor before using antacids. People with kidney failure may develop a build-up of aluminium from these products. This can lead to aluminium toxicity. People with kidney failure also tend to have problems with electrolyte balance. All antacids contain electrolytes, which could make electrolyte balance problems worse.

Object

Evaluate marketed antacid tablets for their release profile

References

1. Applied Biopharmaceutics & Pharmacokinetics, Fifth Edition., Leon Shargel, Susanna Wu-Pong and Andrew Yu
2. Drake D, Hollander D: Neutralizing capacity and cost effectiveness of antacids. Ann Intern Med 1981; 94: 215-217

Requirements

Chemicals: Diazene tablets, Gelucil tablets, Diovol tablets, Univol tablets, Ethanol, 0.1 N HCl, Buffer tablets pH 4 and 1.2.

Glassware: Volumetric flasks, beaker, glass rod, mortar pestle etc.

Principle

Antacids are substances that neutralize stomach acidity. Antacids either directly neutralize acidity, increasing the pH, or reversibly reduce or block the secretion of acid by gastric cells to reduce acidity in the stomach. When gastric hydrochloric acid reaches the nerves in the gastrointestinal mucosa, they signal pain to the central nervous system. This happens when these nerves are exposed. In addition to the reduction of gastric acidity, antacids also alter the profile of prostaglandins produced by gastroduodenal mucosa and this may promote mucosal healing and be related to its therapeutic effects. Antacids are taken by mouth to relieve heartburn, the major symptom of gastroesophageal reflux disease, or acid indigestion. Treatment with antacids alone is symptomatic and only justified for minor symptoms. Side effects from antacids vary depending on the individual, and on other medications they may be taking at the time. Those who experience side effects most commonly suffer from changes in bowel functions, such as diarrhea, constipation, or flatulence.

Tablet antacids are more palatable and portable than liquid antacids and therefore provide a reasonable alternative within a liquid antacid regimen when doses have to be taken outside the home. Because of wide variation in neutralizing ability, the product and the dosage must be known when antacid therapy is being recommended or assessed. These products provide the highest neutralization capacity with the lowest dosage volume, the lowest sodium and calorie contents. Some tablet antacids can be used as alternatives to liquid antacids because of their high neutralization capacity and their portability. Lot-to-lot variability of liquid antacids does exist. It is impossible to predict when such variability will occur, but it may help explain a sudden change in the effectiveness or the ANC of the antacid.

Many new products have been marketed, and the wide variability in Acid Neutralization Capacity (ANC) has been narrowed. Because the efficacy of antacids in reducing gastric acidity is related to their ANC, it is important to know the ANC of currently marketed products.

Procedure

1. Take one tablet each of Gelucil, Diovol, Univol and Diazene and crush them separately in a clean and dried mortar.

2. Take clean and dried 100 mL volumetric flasks and transfer the powdered samples.

3. Moisten with a few drops of ethanol.

4. Make up the volume with 0.1 N HCl.

5. Take a calibrated pH meter and check the pH of the solutions everyone min time interval until a constant reading is obtained.

6. Plot a graph between pH vs time and compare the ANC of the formulations.

Table 1 Acid Neutralizing Capacity of Formulations

Time	pH			
(in mins)	Gelucil	Diazene	Diovol	Univol

Experiment 8

Evaluation of Packaging Material

Pharmaceutical packaging (or drug packaging) is the packages and the packaging processes for pharmaceutical preparations. It involves all of the operations from production through distribution channels to the end consumer. Pharmaceutical packaging is highly regulated but with some variation in the details, depending on the country of origin or the region. Several common factors can include: assurance of patient safety, assurance of the efficacy of the drug through the intended shelf life, uniformity of the drug through different production lots, thorough documentation of all materials and processes, control of possible migration of packaging components into the drug, control of degradation of the drug by oxygen, moisture, heat, etc., prevention of microbial contamination, sterility, etc. Packaging is often involved in dispensing, dosing, and use of the pharmaceutical product. Communication of proper use and cautionary labels are also regulated. Packaging is an integral part of pharmaceutical product.

The packaging materials that are utilised include:

1. Primary Packaging materials: This is the first packaging envelope which is in touch with the dosage form or equipment. The packaging needs to be such that there is no interaction with the drug and will provide proper containment of pharmaceuticals. *E.g*: Blister packages, Strip packages, etc.

2. Secondary Packaging materials: This is consecutive covering or package which stores pharmaceuticals packages in it for their grouping. *E.g.* Cartons, boxes, etc.

3. Tertiary packaging materials: This is to provide bulk handling and shipping of pharmaceuticals from one place to another. *E.g.* Containers, barrels, etc.

The quality of the packaging of pharmaceutical products plays a very important role in the quality of such products. It must: protect against all adverse external influences that can alter the properties of the product, e.g. moisture, light, oxygen and temperature variations; — protect against biological contamination; — protect against physical damage; — carry the correct information and identification of the product. The kind of packaging and the materials used must be chosen in such a way that: — the packaging itself does not have an adverse effect on the product (e.g. through chemical reactions, leaching of packaging materials or absorption); — the product does not have an adverse effect on the packaging, changing its properties or affecting its protective function.

The resulting requirements must be met throughout the whole of the intended shelf-life of the product. Given the link between the quality of a pharmaceutical product and the quality of its packaging, pharmaceutical packaging materials and systems must be subject, in principle, to the same quality assurance requirements as pharmaceutical products.

Object

Evaluate glass as packaging material as per to official standards.

References

1. Indian Pharmacopeia; Volume 1: Government of India Ministry of Health and family welfare; Effective from 1 Aug 2008.

Requirements

Chemicals: Hydrochloric acid, hydrofluoric acid, hydrazine –molybdate, nitric acid, distilled water, methyl red, sulphuric acid, acetone etc.

Glassware: Conical flask, test tube, burette, pipette, glass rod etc.

Apparatus: Autoclave, water bath.

Principle

Glass Containers

Glass containers may be colourless or coloured. Neutral glass is a borosilicate glass containing significant amounts of boric oxide, aluminium oxide, alkali and/or alkaline earth oxides. It has a high hydrolytic resistance and a high thermal shock resistance. Soda-lime-silica glass is a silica glass containing alkali metal oxides, mainly sodium oxide and alkaline earth oxides, mainly calcium oxide. It has only a moderate hydrolytic resistance.

According to their hydrolytic resistance, glass containers are classified as:

- Type I glass containers which are of neutral glass, with a high hydrolytic resistance, suitable for most preparations whether or not for parenteral use,

- Type II glass containers which are usually of soda-lime silica glass with high hydrolytic resistance resulting from suitable treatment of the surface. They are suitable for most acidic and neutral, aqueous preparations whether or not for parenteral use,

- Type III glass containers which are usually of sodalime- silica glass with only moderate hydrolytic resistance. They are generally suitable for non-aqueous preparations for parenteral use, for powders for parenteral use (except for freeze-dried preparations) and for preparations not for parenteral use.

Glass containers intended for parenteral preparations may be ampoules, vials or bottles. The glass used in the manufacture of such containers complies with one of the requirements for hydrolytic resistance given below. Containers of Type II or Type III glass should be used once only. Containers for human blood and blood components must not be re-used. Glass containers with a hydrolytic resistance higher than that recommended for a particular type of preparation may generally also be used. Containers for parenteral preparations are made from uncoloured glass except that coloured glass may be used for substances known to be light - sensitive; in such cases, the containers should be sufficiently transparent to permit visual inspection of the content.

Procedure

Evaluation of glass container as per Indian Pharmacopoeia

Hydrolytic Resistance

Remove any debris or dust from the containers. Rinse each container at least twice with *water* at room temperature. Just before the test rinse each container with freshly prepared *distilled water* and allow to drain.

Complete the cleaning procedure from the first rinsing in not less than 20 minutes and not more than 25 minutes. Fill the containers to the brim with freshly prepared distilled water, empty them and determine the average overflow volume.

Heat closed ampoules on a water-bath or in an air-oven at about 50°. Fill the ampoules with freshly prepared *distilled water* to the maximum volume compatible with sealing them by fusion of the glass and seal them.

Fill bottles or vials to 90 per cent of their calculated overflow volume and cover them with borosilicate glass dishes or aluminium foil previously rinsed with freshly prepared *distilled water*.

Place the containers in an autoclave containing water so that they remain clear of the water. Close the autoclave, displace the air by passage of steam for 10 minutes, raise the temperature from 100° to 121° over

20 minutes, maintain a temperature of 121° for 60 minutes and reduce the temperature from 121° to 100° over 40 minutes, venting to prevent vacuum. Remove the containers from the autoclave and cool them in a bath of running tap water.

Carry out the following titration within 1 hour of removing the containers from the autoclave. Combine the liquids from the containers under examination, measure the volume of test solution specified into a conical flask and add 0.15 ml of *methyl red solution* for each 50 mL of liquid.

Titrate with 0.01M hydrochloric acid taking as the end-point the colour obtained by repeating the operation using the same volume of freshly prepared *distilled water*.

The difference between the preparations represents the volume of 0.01M hydrochloric acid required by the test solution calculate the volume of 0.01M hydrochloric acid required for each mL of test solution, if necessary. The result is not greater than the value stated.

Test for arsenic

Prepare a test solution as described in the test for Hydrolytic resistance for an adequate number of ampoules to produce 50mL. Pipette 10 mL of the test solution from the combined contents of all the ampoules into a flask, add 10 mL of nitric acid and evaporate to dryness on a water-bath.

Dry the residue in an oven at 130° for 30 minutes. Cool, add to the residue 10.0 mL of hydrazine-molybdate reagent, swirl to dissolve and heat under reflux on a water-bath for 20 minutes. Cool to room temperature.

Determine the absorbance of the resulting solution at the maximum at about 840nm (2.4.7), using 10.0 mL of hydrazine-molybdate reagent as the blank.

The absorbance of the test solution does not exceed the absorbance obtained by repeating the determination using 0.1 mL of arsenic standard solution (10 ppm As) in place of the test solution (0.1 ppm)

Evaluation of glass container as per United States Pharmacopoeia.

Powdered Glass Test

Rinse thoroughly with purified water six or more containers selected at random, and dry them with a current of clean, dry air. Crush the containers into fragments about 25 mm in size, divide about 100 g of the coarsely crushed glass into three approximately equal portions, and place one of the portions in the special mortar.

With the pestle in place, crush the glass further by striking 3 or 4 blows with the hammer. Nest the sieves and empty the mortar into the No. 20 sieve. Repeat the operation on each of the two remaining portions of glass, emptying the mortar each time into the No. 20 sieve. Shake the sieves for a short time, then remove the glass from the Nos. 20 and 40 sieves, and again crush and sieve as before.

Repeat again this crushing and sieving operation. Empty the receiving pan, reassemble the nest of sieves, and shake by mechanical means for 5 minutes or by hand for an equivalent length of time. Transfer the portion retained on the No. 50 sieve, which should weigh in excess of 10 g, to a closed container, and store in a desiccator until used for the test.

Spread the specimen on a piece of glazed paper and pass a magnet through it to remove particles of iron that may be introduced during the crushing. Transfer the specimen to a 250-mL conical flask of resistant glass and wash it with six 30mL portions of acetone, swirling each time for about 30 seconds, and carefully decanting the acetone. After washing, the specimen should be free from agglomerations of glass powder, and the surface of the grains should be practically free from adhering fine particles. Dry the flask and contents for 20 minutes at 140, transfer the grains to a weighing bottle, and cool in a desiccator. Use the test specimen within 48 hours after drying.

Transfer 10.00 g of the prepared specimen, accurately weighed, to a 250mL conical flask that has been digested (aged) previously with high-purity water in a bath at 90 for at least 24 hours or at 121 for 1 hour.

Add 50.0 mL of high-purity water to this flask and to one similarly prepared to provide a blank. Cap all flasks with borosilicate glass beakers that previously have been treated as described for the flasks and that are of such size that the bottoms of the beakers fit snugly down on the top rims of the containers.

Place the containers in the autoclave, and close it securely, leaving the vent cock open. Heat until steam issues vigorously from the vent cock and continue heating for 10 minutes. Close the vent cock, and adjust the temperature to 121, taking 19 to 23 minutes to reach the desired temperature.

Hold the temperature at 121 ± 2.0 for 30 minutes, counting from the time this temperature is reached. Reduce the heat so that the autoclave cools and comes to atmospheric pressure in 38 to 46 minutes, being vented as necessary to prevent the formation of a vacuum.

Cool the flask at once in running water, decant the water from the flask into a suitably cleansed vessel, and wash the residual powdered glass with four 15-mL portions of High-Purity Water, adding the decanted washings to the main portion.

Add 5 drops of Methyl Red Solution and titrate immediately with 0.020 N sulfuric acid. If the volume of titrating solution is expected to be less than 10 mL, use a microburet. Record the volume of 0.020 N sulfuric acid used to neutralize the extract from 10 g of the prepared specimen of glass, corrected for a blank. The volume does not exceed that indicated in Table 1 for the type of glass concerned.

Table 1 Test Limits for Powdered Glass Test

Type	General Description a	Type of Test	Size, b mL	Limits mL of 0.020 N Acid
I	Highly resistant, borosilicate glass	Powdered Glass	All	1.0
III	Soda-lime glass	Powdered Glass	All	8.5
a. The description applies to containers of this type of glass usually available.				
b. Size indicates the overflow capacity of the container.				

Water Attack at 121

Rinse thoroughly 3 or more containers, selected at random, twice with High-Purity Water. Fill each container to 90% of its overflow capacity with High-Purity Water, and proceed as directed for Procedure under Powdered Glass Test, beginning with "Cap all flasks," except that the time of autoclaving shall be 60 minutes instead of 30 minutes, and ending with "to prevent the formation of a vacuum."

Empty the contents from 1 or more containers into a 100mL graduated cylinder, combining, in the case of smaller containers, the contents of several containers to obtain a volume of 100mL.

Place the pooled specimen in a 250mL conical flask of resistant glass, add 5 drops of Methyl Red Solution, and titrate, while warm, with 0.020 N sulfuric acid. Complete the titration within 60 minutes after opening the autoclave.

Record the volume of 0.020 N sulfuric acid used, corrected for a blank obtained by titrating 100 mL of high-purity water at the same temperature and with the same amount of indicator. The volume does not exceed that indicated in Table 2.

Table 2 Test Limit for Water Attack at 121

Type	General Description a	Type of Test	Limits	
			Size, b mL	mL of 0.020 N Acid
II	Treated soda-lime glass	Water Attack	100 or less	0.7
			Over 100	0.2

a. The description applies to containers of this type of glass usually available.
b. Size indicates the overflow capacity of the container.

Arsenic

Arsenic 211 — Use as the Test Preparation 35 mL of the water from one Type I glass container or, in the case of smaller containers, 35 mL of the combined contents of several Type I glass containers, prepared as directed for procedure under water attack at 121 or surface glass test: the limit is 0.1 µg per g.

Experiment 9

Estimation of Pharmacokinetic Parameters

Pharmacokinetics describe what the body does to the drug, as opposed to pharmacodynamics which describe what the drug does to the body. Pharmacokinetic information is required to optimize the pharmacodynamic response. The primary pharmacokinetic disposition parameter is clearance. Knowledge of this value and its major constituent parts, i.e. fractional renal and hepatic elimination, allows the clinician to prescribe the correct dosage regimen to obtain a mean therapeutic concentration and to predict the effects of various disease states. The other primary disposition parameter, volume of distribution at steady-state, may also vary with changes in physiologic and pathologic conditions. Both clearance and volume of distribution as well as the correlation of concentration measurements with pharmacodynamics would be expected to vary with changes in plasma protein binding. Although plasma concentration measurements are usually easiest to perform, interpretation of parameters in physiologic terms requires blood concentration, so the blood/plasma partition parameter should be determined. Although half-life is a composite parameter reflecting changes in both clearance and volume of distribution, it is a value which defines the maximum and minimum blood concentrations obtained for a particular dosage regimen, important quantities in defining the pharmacodynamic response. The major pharmacokinetic input parameter is the extent of availability as a function of route of administration. This parameter, as well as all of the disposition parameters discussed above, may be determined without designating a particular pharmacokinetic model. Only the rate of availability requires a model, although peak time and peak concentration are reasonable noncompartmental substitutes.

Pharmacokinetic parameters are assessed by monitoring variations in concentration of the drug and/or its metabolites in physiological fluids that are easy to access (i.e., plasma and urine). Plasma concentrations are usually checked, and in addition biopsies can be taken from animals and sometimes from humans. Pharmacokinetic parameters give an overall indication of the behavior of the drug in the body. Since the kinetics of absorption, distribution, metabolism, and excretion of a drug are usually linear, a polyexponential function may be adjusted to the plasma concentrations allowing the calculation of pharmacokinetic parameters. However, adjustment is not always feasible and is not mandatory. It is sufficient to consider the terminal part of the concentrations-versus-time curve, assuming that absorption and distribution, being almost complete, would have no significant influence on both metabolism and excretion. Pharmacokinetics of a drug depends on patient-related factors as well as on the drug's chemical properties.

Object

Solve the given data for the estimation of pharmacokinetic parameters

Requirements

Graph paper, Scale etc.

References

1. Biopharmaceutics and Pharmacokinetics by By Brahmankar DM, Jaiswal SB Publisher: Vallabh Prakashan

2. Applied Biopharmaceutics & Pharmacokinetics, Fifth Edition., Leon Shargel, Susanna Wu-Pong and Andrew Yu.

Principle

Pharmacokinetics, is a branch of pharmacology dedicated to the determination of the fate of substances administered externally to a living organism. The substances of interest include pharmaceutical agents, hormones, nutrients, and toxins. Pharmacokinetics is divided into several areas including the extent and rate of absorption, distribution, metabolism and excretion. This is commonly referred to as the ADME scheme:

1. Absorption - the process of a substance entering the blood circulation.

2. Distribution - the dispersion or dissemination of substances throughout the fluids and tissues of the body.

3. Metabolism (or Biotransformation) - the irreversible transformation of parent compounds into daughter metabolites.

4. Excretion - the removal of the substances from the body. In rare cases, some drugs irreversibly accumulate in body tissue.

Elimination is the result of metabolism and excretion. Pharmacokinetics describes how the body affects a specific drug after administration. Pharmacokinetic properties of drugs may be affected by elements such as the site of administration and the dose of administered drug. These may affect the absorption rate.

The following are the most commonly measured pharmacokinetic metrics:

Characteristic	Description	Abbreviation(s)	Formula
Dose	Loading dose (LD), or maintenance dose (MD).	D	design parameter
T	Dosing interval.	τ	design parameter
Volume of distribution	The apparent volume in which a drug is distributed	Vd	D/C0
Concentration	Amount of drug in a given volume of plasma.	C0 or Css	$= D/V_d$
Elimination half-life	The time required for the concentration of the drug to reach half of its original value.	$t_{1/2}$	$= ln(2)/k_e$
Elimination rate constant	The rate at which drugs are removed from the body.	k_e	$= ln(2)/t_{1/2} =$ CL/V_d
Elimination rate	Rate of infusion required to balance elimination.	k_{in}	$= C_{ss}.CL$
Area under the curve	The integral of the concentration-time curve (after a single dose or in steady state).	$AUC_{0-\infty}$ $AUC_{\tau,ss}$	$= \int_0^\infty C\, dt$ $= \int_t^{t+\tau} C\, dt$
Clearance	The volume of plasma cleared of the drug per unit time.	CL	$= V_d \cdot k_e =$ D/AUC
Bioavailability	The systemically available fraction of a drug.	f	$\dfrac{AUC_{po}.D_{iv}}{AUC_{iv}.D_{po}}$
C_{max}	The peak plasma concentration of a drug after administration.	C_{max}	direct measurement
t_{max}	Time to reach C_{max}.	t_{max}	direct measurement
C_{min}	The lowest (trough) concentration that a drug reaches before the next dose is administered.	$C_{min,ss}$	direct measurement

Numericals

1. A 60 kg male received an antibiotic at a dose of 2mg/kg orally. Assuming one compartment open model kinetics, calculate elimination rate constant, biological half-life, volume of distribution and AUC from the given data.

Time in hrs	Plasma drug concentration in µg/mL
0	0.00
0.25	2.2
0.5	3.8
075	5.0

Table *Contd..*

Time in hrs	Plasma drug concentration in µg/mL
1.0	5.8
1.5	6.8
2.0	7.1
2.5	7.1
3	6.9
4	6.2
6	4.8
8	3.5
12	1.9
18	0.8
24	0.3

2. Calculate $t_{1/2}$, K_e, C_0 and V_d from the given data, when an IV bolus administration of a 400 mg of dose was given and it followed one compartment kinetics.

Plasma Drug Concentration µg/ml	Time hr	Log C
88.4	0.5	1.944
74.0	1.0	1.869
50.0	2.0	1.699
38.5	3.0	1.585
26.0	5.0	1.415
21.8	7.0	1.388

3. A single dose of a drug was given to a 70 kg patient at a dose of 10 mg/kg. Urine samples were collected periodically. Calculate various pharmacokinetic parameters using the given data.

Time of urine collection 't' (hr)	Volume of urine collected (mL)	Concentration of unchanged drug in urine (µg/mL)
2	120	1200
4	170	600
6	130	530
8	240	200
12	240	190
24	900	40

4. If plasma concentration of a drug after IV bolus dose of 300 mg was found to be 10 and 5.5 µg/mL at 2 and 4 hrs respectively, assuming one compartment kinetics, calculate half-life of drug and total clearance.

5. A drug was administered at a dose of 500 mg to a healthy male volunteer. Determine the plasma drug concentration at 4 hrs when

volume of distribution if 30 litres and elimination half-life is given to be 0.2 hrs.

6. Calculate MRT and average V_d at steady state when the drug is given as IV bolus at a dose of 100 mg. Given $K_e = 0.017$/hrs, AUC= 55.32 and AUMC = 66.19.

7. AUC values of penicillin upon 50 mg of IV administration and 100 mg of oral administration were found to be 70 and 90 respectively. Calculate absolute bioavailability of penicillin and relative bioavailability of penicillin from tablet based on penicillin suspension whose dose is 100 mg and AUC is 95.

8. A new drug was given as IV bolus of 300 mg to a healthy volunteer weighing 80 kgs. Immediately after injection, the blood level was found to be 3.75 mg/100mL. After 6 hrs, it was 2.2 mg/100mL. Calculate plasma elimination rate constant.

9. A drug has elimination half-life of 8 hrs and follows one compartment kinetics. If a single dose of 250 mg is given to an adult male volunteer weighing 68 kgs by IV bolus, calculate % drug lost in 48 hrs.

10. Determine oral bioavailability of the given drug/formulation by urinary excretion method using animal model.

Table 1

S. No	Time in hrs Dt	Absorbance in nm	Concentration (µg/mL)	Volume of urine (mL) Du	Concentration of drug in urine (mg)	Du/Dt	log Du/Dt	t*
1	0.25	1.105	30	715				
2	0.50	1.705	20	695				
3	1.0	1.278	55	635				
4	2.0	1.505	65	600				
5	4.0	1.562	44	375				
6	6.0	0.296	26	125				

A subject received a single IV dose of a drug solution containing 100 mg of the drug. The plasma drug concentration was obtained as given in the table. Calculate,

1. Values for α and β,

2. half-life for the distributive phase and the elimination phase,

3. Give equation and calculate concentration of drug 9.5hr after administration.

4. Volume of distribution of the central compartment,

5. Fraction of the drug in the central compartment in the post distributive phase,

6. Values of k12, k21 and k,

7. AUC,

8. Assume that drug follows two compartment model.

Time (hr)	Plasma Drug Concentration (μg/mL)	log C
0.5	7.78	0.891
1	6.4	0.806
1.5	5.51	0.741
2	4.91	0.691
2.5	4.89	0.689
3	4.17	0.620
4	3.7	0.568
5	3.35	0.525
6	3.05	0.484
8	2.54	0.405
10	2.12	0.326
12	1.77	0.248
14	1.48	0.170

Estimation of Pharmacokinetic Parameters by Urinary Excretion Method

The study of the excretion of a drug and its metabolites in urine after drug administration can provide valuable information concerning drug absorption, distribution and elimination. The maximum value of these studies is, however, only obtained by a detailed kinetic analysis of the experimental results. While certain procedures may be preferable for a specific purpose, two methods of treating the experimental results are capable of general application and are suitable for mathematical interpretation. The first is derived from the classical method of chemical kinetics. In principle it seeks to calculate the amount of drug in the body from a knowledge of the amount of drug excreted at that time and the total amount finally excreted. Its application to drug urinary excretion data will here be termed the "Sigma-minus" method. The second is the "Rate" method. This is based on a study of the decline in the rate of excretion of drug in the urine. After the oral administration of a drug, there is an initial period when absorption is in progress. Any drug which is subsequently absorbed but which at that time is in the gastrointestinal tract is interpreted in this plot as present in the body, so that in the present context the meaning of the plot during this period is fictional. Subsequently, when absorption of drug has ceased or has become negligible, a plot which is based on the unchanged drug in urine represents the decline of that fraction of the total drug in the body which ultimately appears in the urine as unchanged drug. When drug elimination is first order, K may be determined from the slope of the terminal, linear section of the log "Sigma-minus" plot.

When drug elimination is first order and the process of drug absorption has ceased, a log plot of the rate of excretion of drug against time exhibits a terminal linear section of slope equal to $-K$. In addition to those factors which govern its formation, the excretion of a metabolite in urine is governed by an elimination rate constant which consists of a rate constant for its urinary excretion and the rate constants for its elimination by other routes-for example, by further metabolism. The following considerations relate to a metabolite which is eliminated only by urinary excretion, in this instance therefore its rate of elimination is governed only by an excretion rate constant, K_u.

The rate constants governing metabolite formation also constitute the only valid basis for the comparison of the rate of metabolism of drugs.

This method of assessing bioavailability is based on the principle that the urinary excretion of unchanged drug is directly proportional to the plasma concentration of drug. The study is particularly useful for drugs extensively excreted unchanged in urine for ex; certain thiazide diuretics and sulfonamides and for drugs that have urine as the site of action.

Object

Calculate pharmacokinetic parameters using urinary excretion method for the drug Diclofenac sodium.

References

1. Cummings, A. J., King, M. L. & Martin, B. K. (1967). A kinetic study of drug elimination based on the excretion of paracetamol and its metabolites in man. Br. J. Pharmac. Chemother., 29, 150-157.

2. Wagner, J. G. (1963). Some possible errors in the plotting and interpretation of semilogarithmic plots of blood level and urinary excretion data. J. Pharm. Sci., 52, 1097-1 101.

Requirements

Chemicals: Diclofenac sodium, Potable water, Buffer tablet pH 7.4

Glassware: Beaker (250 ml), Measuring cylinder, Glass rod, Volumetric flask (100 ml)

Principle

The study of the excretion of a drug and its metabolites in urine after drug administration can provide valuable information concerning drug absorption, distribution and elimination. The maximum value of these studies is, however, only obtained by a detailed kinetic analysis of the experimental results. While certain procedures may be preferable for a specific purpose, two methods of treating the experimental results are capable of general application and are suitable for mathematical interpretation. The first is derived from the classical method of chemical kinetics. In principle it seeks to calculate the amount of drug in the body from a knowledge of the amount of drug excreted at that time and the total amount finally excreted. Its application to drug urinary excretion data will here be termed the "Sigma-minus" method. The second is the "Rate" method. This is based on a study of the decline in the rate of excretion of drug in the urine. These methods cannot, however, be regarded simply as alternative procedures. They do not necessarily provide identical information, and each method can on certain occasions yield information which is not available from the other.

Application to the excretion of drug in urine

(i) The " Sigma-minus" method

This method was used by Bray, Thorpe & White (1951). When applied to the excretion of unchanged drug in urine the " Sigma-minus " method consists of plotting log (Dc,-Du) against time, where (Du, -Du) represents the sum (Sigma) of the amounts of drug excreted until such time as excretion may be considered to be complete (Du00) minus the cumulative amount of drug excreted to a time t, (Do). When drug elimination is first order, this is based on the equation:

$$\text{In } (Du \, x - Du) = \text{In } kd \, Do - Kt \qquad \text{.....(1)}$$

D'. is a constant which may be interpreted as that amount of drug which if present in the body at t = o would ultimately give rise to a pattern of drug decline identical to that observed on this occasion after the administration of the dose Do. The slope of the plot is equal to -K.

After the oral administration of a drug there is an initial period when absorption is in progress. Any drug which is subsequently absorbed but which at that time is in the gastrointestinal tract is interpreted in this plot as present in the body, so that in the present context the meaning of the plot during this period is fictional. Subsequently, when absorption of drug has ceased or has become negligible, a plot which is based on the unchanged drug in urine represents the decline of that fraction of the total drug in the body which ultimately appears in the urine as unchanged drug (equation (1)). When drug elimination is first order, K may be determined from the slope of the terminal, linear section of the log "Sigma-minus" plot. Reference to this method as a plot of the log "amount of drug in the body" or log "amount not yet excreted" can for the above reasons be misleading, and it will be shown to be particularly so when applied to a metabolite. The nomenclature "Sigma-minus" provides a simple description which avoids these implications and describes the method in terms only of the method of calculation. The "Sigma-minus" method requires knowledge of D, o and in theory therefore requires the collection of urine until such time as excretion is complete. In practice, urine is collected over a number of consecutive short intervals of time and then over one or more longer periods until the drug can no longer be estimated. Wagner (1963) has suggested that the collection of urine for a period corresponding to 10 half-lives of the drug is usually adequate for this purpose. He also emphasized that failure to determine or use the true recovery value can give rise to curvature in the plot. The examination of a number of theoretical plots shows, however, that a small error in the assessment of Du, can give rise to plots which could well be interpreted as linear over a considerable period, but that the slope of the apparently linear section then shows an appreciable departure from the true slope. In practice, such an interpretation is even more likely, for analytical errors frequently accompanied by actual fluctuations in the rate of drug elimination, will also operate to give departure from perfect linearity.

Procedure

1. Select normal male volunteers and fast overnight.
2. Administer 200 mL of cold purified water and collect the first urine sample.
3. Name it as blank.
4. Selected volunteers were administered tablet with 200 mL of cold potable water.
5. Collect urine samples at regular time intervals. Encourage full bladder emptying during each collection.
6. Observe the absorbance after proper dilution of the urine with suitable dilution media.
7. Plot graph taking logDu/ Dt vs t* and cumulative amount excreted (mg) in Y-axis and time (hrs) in X axis.
8. Calculate the parameters.

Table 1

Time interval (hr)	Urine volume (mL)	Urine concentration (mg/mL)	Amount excreted ΔU (mg)	Cumulative amount excreted U (mg)	Mid point time T_{midpt} (hr)	Rate of excretion ΔU/Δt (mg/hr)	A.R.E (mg)
0-2							
2-4							
4-6							
6-8							
8-10							
10-12							
12-18							
18-24							
24-∞							

Experiment 11

Estimation of Protein Binding

Many drugs interact with plasma or tissue proteins or with other macromolecules, such as melanin and DNA, to form a drug–macromolecule complex. The formation of a drug protein complex is often named drug–protein binding. The more blood volume the organ has, the faster the amount of drug diffused. Then, there occurs redistribution of drugs in some organs. e.g. Thiopental is lipophilic drug, and it diffuses into brain more quickly, then, redistribute to the fat and other tissues. The concentration of drug at target organ should be measured through the concentration of plasma. So, the effect of the drug may be estimated at target organ. Protein binding describes the ability of proteins to form bonds with other substances, and most commonly refers to the bonding of drugs to these molecules in blood plasma, red blood cells, other components of the blood, and to tissue membranes.

The binding of drug to plasma (and tissue) proteins is a major determinant of drug disposition (distribution). Binding has a very important effect on drug dynamics since only the free (unbound) drug interacts with receptors. The proteins commonly involved in binding with drugs are albumin, lipoproteins, and a1-acid-glycoprotein (AGP). Acidic and neutral compounds will tend to bond with albumin, which is basic, while basic substances will primarily bind to the acidic AGP molecule.

The bound drug is kept in the blood stream while the unbound component may be metabolized or excreted, making it the active part. So, if a drug is 95% bound to a binding protein and 5% is free, that means that 5% is active in the system and causing pharmacological effects. Drug–protein binding may be a reversible or an irreversible process.

- Irreversible drug–protein binding is usually a result of chemical activation of the drug, which then attaches strongly to the protein or macromolecule by covalent chemical bonding. For example, the hepatotoxicity of high doses of acetaminophen is due to the formation of reactive metabolite intermediates that interact with liver proteins.

- Reversible drug–protein binding implies that the drug binds the protein with weaker chemical bonds, such as hydrogen bonds or Vander Waals forces.

A drug's efficiency may be affected by the degree to which it binds to the proteins within blood plasma. The less bound a drug is, the more efficiently it can traverse cell membranes or diffuse. Common blood proteins that drugs bind to are human serum albumin, lipoprotein, glycoprotein, α, β, and γ globulins.

Object

Study protein binding characteristics of the given drug Paracetamol

References

1. Forrest JA, Clements JA, Prescott LF. Clinical pharmacokinetics of paracetamol. Clin Pharmacokin. 1982; 7: 93-107.
2. Shek KLA, Chan LN, Nutescu E. Warfarin acetaminophen drug interaction revisited. Pharmacotherapy 1999; 19: 1153–58.

Requirements

Chemicals: Paracetamol pure drug, tryptophan, Egg albumin, Egg membrane or any other semi permeable membrane, di sodium hydrogen ortho phosphate, potassium di hydrogen ortho phosphate and sodium chloride.

Glassware: Beaker (250 mL), Measuring cylinder, Glass rod, Mortar Pestle, Volumetric flask (10 and 100 mL), Watch Glass.

Principle

The rate of absorption of oral paracetamol depends on the rate of gastric emptying and is usually rapid and complete. The mean systemic availability is about 75%. Paracetamol is extensively metabolized, and the plasma half-life is 1.5-2.5 hours. About 55% and 30% of a therapeutic dose is excreted in the urine as glucuronide and sulphate conjugates, respectively, whereas mercapturic acid and cysteine conjugates (representing conversion to a potentially toxic intermediate metabolite) each account for some 4% of the dose. Paracetamol metabolism is age and dose dependent. With hepatotoxic doses, paracetamol metabolism is impaired and the half-life prolonged. Sulphate conjugation is saturated, and the proportion excreted as mercapturic acid and cysteine conjugates is increased. The renal clearance of paracetamol depends on urine flow rate by not pH. The renal clearances of the glucuronide and sulphate conjugates often exceed the glomerular filtration rate and are independent of urine flow and pH. Acetaminophen sulfate is greater than 50% protein bound, as determined by equilibrium dialysis and ultrafiltration. There is a limited amount of data on the binding of paracetamol to plasma proteins. In therapeutic doses paracetamol is a safe analgesic, but in overdosage it can cause severe hepatic necrosis. Following oral administration, it is rapidly absorbed from the gastro-intestinal tract, its systemic bioavailability being dose-dependent and ranging from 70 to 90%. Its rate of oral absorption is predominantly dependent on the rate of gastric emptying, being delayed by food, propantheline, pethidine and diamorphine and enhanced by metoclopramide. Paracetamol is also well absorbed from the rectum. It distributes rapidly and evenly throughout most tissues and fluids and has a volume of distribution of approximately 0.9L/kg. 10 to 20% of the drug is bound to red blood cells. Paracetamol is extensively metabolised (predominantly in the liver), the major metabolites being the sulphate and glucuronide conjugates. A minor fraction of drug is converted to a highly reactive alkylating metabolite which is inactivated with reduced glutathione and excreted in the urine as cysteine and mercapturic acid conjugates. Large doses of paracetamol (overdoses) cause acute hepatic necrosis as a result of depletion of glutathione and of binding of the excess reactive metabolite to vital cell constituents. This damage can be prevented by the early administration of sulfhydryl compounds such as methionine and N-acetylcysteine. In healthy subjects 85 to 95% of a therapeutic dose is excreted in the urine within 24 hours with about 4, 55, 30, 4 and 4% appearing as unchanged paracetamol and its glucuronide, sulphate, mercapturic acid and cysteine conjugates, respectively. The plasma half-life in such subjects ranges from 1.9 to 2.5 hours and the total body clearance from 4.5 to 5.5 mL/kg/min. Age has little effect on the plasma half-life, which is shortened in patients taking anticonvulsants. The plasma half-life is usually normal in patients with mild chronic liver disease, but its prolonged in those with decompensated liver disease. It has been suggested that binding might influence the ability of some analytical methods to quantify the total amount of drug present in the plasma fraction, the basis of clinical experience in risk assessment and antidote usage.

The present experiment deals with studying the protein binding effects of paracetamol using egg albumin as the protein. The rate kinetics involved in the study of drug-protein binding can be understood through Michaelis-Menton equation.

$$V = d[p] / dt$$

$$= V_{max} = [S] / K_m + [S]$$

Where,

V = rate of reaction

[S] = concentration of substrate

K_m = Michaelis constant

V_{max} = maximum rate achieved by the system at saturating substrate concentrations

Procedure

1. Prepare 800 mL of Phosphate Buffer saline 7.4.
2. Take an egg and separate the albumin part from it and measure it.
3. Take a 25 mL volumetric flask and transfer 100 mg of accurately weighed quantity of drug.
4. Dissolve the drug in 10 mL of buffer and make up the volume with PBS 7.4.
5. In another 25 mL volumetric flask, take 100 mg of accurately weighed amount of the drug, add 10 mL of PBS 7.4, dissolve the drug and then add 10 mL of albumin to it. Mix thoroughly.
6. Make up the volume with PBS 7.4.
7. Take these mixtures separately into semi-permeable membranes which is fixed to diffusion tubes and dip into 100 mL of PBS 7.4 solution which maintained at 37±0.5°C.
8. Stir the system at 75 rpm using magnetic stirrer.
9. Collect 5 mL of aliquots at regular intervals and replace with fresh pre-warmed PBS 7.4.
10. Continue the study for 8 hrs and analyse the samples spcctrophotometrically at 257 nm.
11. After 5 hrs tryptophan was added to the mixture. As the binding sites of these drugs are same, therefore the replacement concentration was analysed.

Preparation of calibration curve of paracetamol: Dissolve 100 mg of Paracetamol in PBS 7.4 in a 100 mL of volumetric flask. Treat this as stock solution. Dilute this stock solution suitably to get concentrations 1,2,3,4,5,6,7,8,9 and 10 µg/mL. Measure absorbance at 257 nm and plot calibration curve taking concentration (µg/mL) on x axis and absorbance on y axis. Derive regression equation.

Calculate concentration of drug released at regular intervals and determine cumulative drug released. Plot a graph taking time on x axis and cumulative drug released on y axis.

Report the effect of binding on the release pattern/behaviour of Paracetamol.

Table 1

S. No.	Time in min	Absorbance	Concentration (X) µg/mL	(X × 5) µg/mL	(X × 100) µg/mL	Cumulative amount of drug released µg
0	0					
1	30					
2	60					
3	90					
4	120					
5	150					
6	180					

Experiment 12

Bioequivalence Study of Paracetamol

Bioequivalence is a term in pharmacokinetics used to assess the expected *in vivo* biological equivalence of two proprietary preparations of a drug. If two products are said to be bioequivalent it means that they would be expected to be, for all intents and purposes, the same. Pharmaceutical equivalence implies the same amount of the same active substance(s), in the same dosage form, for the same route of administration and meeting the same or comparable standards.

In determining bioequivalence, for example, between two products such as a commercially available Brand product and a potential to-be-marketed Generic product, pharmacokinetic studies are conducted whereby each of the preparations are administered in a cross-over study to volunteer subjects, generally healthy individuals but occasionally in patients.

Serum/plasma samples are obtained at regular intervals and assayed for parent drug (or occasionally metabolite) concentration. Occasionally, blood concentration levels are neither feasible or possible to compare the two products (e.g. inhaled corticosteroids), then pharmacodynamic endpoints rather than pharmacokinetic endpoints (see below) are used for comparison. For a pharmacokinetic comparison, the plasma concentration data are used to assess key pharmacokinetic parameters such as area under the curve (AUC), peak concentration (C_{max}), time to peak concentration (T_{max}), and absorption lag time (t_{lag}). Testing should be conducted at several different doses, especially when the drug displays non-linear pharmacokinetics.

Object

Perform bioequivalence studies of different brand of Paracetamol.

References

1. Shargel S., Wu pangs; applied biopharmaceutics & pharmacokinetics, 5th edition. Indian Pharmacopoeia edition 2007.

Theory

Bioequivalence is a term in pharmacokinetics used to assess the expected *in vivo* biological of two proprietary preparations of drug. If two products are said to be bioequivalent it means that they would be expected to be, for all intents and purposes, the same.

In determining bioequivalence, for example, between two products such as a commercially-available Brand product and a potential to-be-marketed Generic product, pharmacokinetic studies are conducted whereby each of the preparations are administered in a cross-over study to volunteer subjects, generally healthy individuals but occasionally in patients. Serum/plasma samples are obtained at a regular interval and assayed for parent drug (or occasionally metabolite) concentration. Occasionally, blood concentration levels are neither feasible nor possible to compare the two products (e.g. inhaled corticosteroids), then pharmacodynamic endpoints rather than pharmacokinetic endpoints (see below) are used for comparison. For a pharmacokinetic comparison, the plasma concentration data are used to assess key pharmacokinetic parameters such as area under the curve (AUC), peak concentration (C_{max}), time to peak concentration (T_{max}), and absorption lag time (t_{lag}). Testing should be conducted at several different doses, especially when the drug displays non-linear pharmacokinetics.

In addition to data from bioequivalence studies, other data may need to be submitted to meet regulatory requirements for bioequivalence. Such evidence may include:

- Analytical method validation

- *In-vitro in –vivo* correlation studies

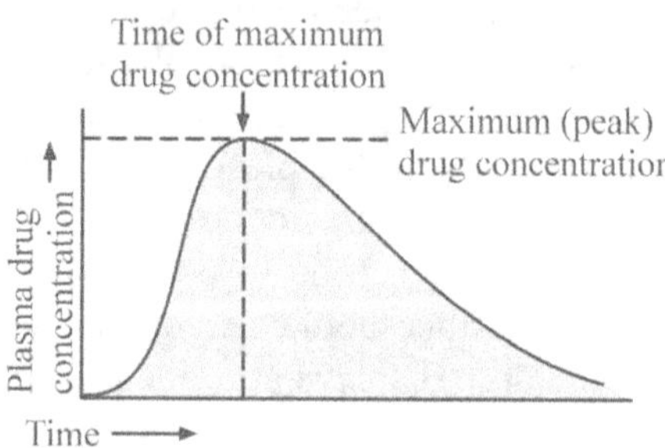

Bioequivalent drug products, this term describes pharmaceutical equivalent or pharmaceutical alternative products that display comparable bioavailability when studied under similar experimental conditions. For systemically absorbed drugs, the test (generic) and reference listed drug (brand-name) shall be considered bioequivalent if: (1) the rate and extent of absorption of the drug do not show a significant difference from the rate and extent of absorption of the reference drug when administered at the same molar dose of the therapeutic ingredient under similar experimental conditions in either a single dose or multiple doses; or (2) the extent of absorption of the test drug does not show a significant difference from the extent of absorption of the reference drug when administered at the same M in molar dose of the therapeutic ingredient under similar experiment conditions in either a single dose or multiple doses.

Bioavailability studied are performed for both approved active drug ingredients and therapeutic moieties not yet approved for marketing by the FDA. New formulations of active drug ingredients must be approved by FDA before marketing, the FDA ensures that the drug product is safe and effective for its labeled indication for use; moreover, the drug product must meet all applicable standards of identity strength, quality, & purity.

Bioequivalence of different formulations of the same drug substance in values equivalence with respect to rate & extent of systemic drug absorption, clinical interpretation is important in evaluating the result of a bioequivalence study.

A small difference between drugs products, even if statistically significant may produce very little difference in therapeutic response. Generally, two formulations are considered that the difference of less than 20% in AUC and C_{max} between drug products is unlikely to be clinically significant in patient. The task for further stated that clinical studies of effectiveness have difficulty detecting difference in the doses Tween 50 and 100%, therefore normal variation is observed in medical practice and plasma drug level may vary among individuals greater than 20%.

Paracetamol IP Monograph

Description: White crystals or a white crystalline powder.

The tablet of paracetamol must not contain less than 95% and not more than 105%.

Solubility: Soluble in ethanol 95% and acetone sparingly soluble ether, very slightly soluble in Dichloromethane.

Dissolution

Medium: 900 mL of phosphate buffer pH 5.8

Speed of time: 50rpm and 30 minutes

Withdraw a suitable volume of the medium and filtrate with the same solvent measure about 275nm. Similarly, measure the absorbance of the solution of known concentration of paracetamol. Calculate the content of the paracetamol.

Not less than 80% of the started amount of paracetamol.

Assay: Weigh and power 20 tablets. Weigh accurately a quantity of a powder containing about 0.15g of paracetamol and 50mL of 0.1M sodium hydroxide dilute with 100mL of water, shake for 15min and add sufficient water to produce 200mL. Mix, filter and dilute 10.0mL of the filtrate to 100.0mL with water and mix. Measure the absorbance of the resulting solution at about 275nm. Calculate the content of paracetamol.

Procedure

1. Measurement of hardness &friability was done by using Monsanto hardness tester & Roche friabilator respectively.

2. Disintegration time of tablet was observed in 0.1N HCl.

3. Dissolution study of tablet was done by using USP paddle type apparatus in buffer of pH7.8 and at 50 rpm.

Observation

Table 1 Hardness

S. No.	Brand name	A	B	C	Mean hardness
1					
2					
3					
4					
5					

Table 2 Friability

S. No.	Brand Name	% Friability
1		
2		
3		
4		
5		

Table 3 Disintegration

S. No.	Brand Name	Disintegration Time
1		
2		
3		
4		
5		

Table 4 Drug Release Profile of Brand 1

S. No	Time in mins	Absorbance in nm	Concentration (c) µg/mL	(c × 0.5) µg/mL	(c × 30) µg/mL	CDR	% CDR	Log CDR
1	0							
2	15							
3	30							
4	60							
5	90							
6	120							
7	150							
8	180							
9	210							
10	240							
11	300							
12	360							
13	390							
14	420							
15	480							

Table 5 Drug Release Profile of Brand 2

S. No.	Time in mins	Absorbance in nm	Concentration (c)µg/mL	(c × 0.5) µg/mL	(c × 30) µg/mL	CDR	% CDR	Log CDR
1	0							
2	15							
3	30							
4	60							
5	90							
6	120							
7	150							
8	180							
9	210							
10	240							
11	300							
12	360							
13	390							
14	420							
15	480							

Table 6 Drug Release Profile of Brand 3

S. No.	Time in mins	Absorbance in nm	Concentration (c)µg/mL	(c × 0.5) µg/mL	(c × 30) µg/mL	CDR	% CDR	Log CDR
1	0							
2	15							
3	30							
4	60							
5	90							
6	120							
7	150							
8	180							
9	210							
10	240							
11	300							
12	360							
13	390							
14	420							
15	480							

Table 7 Drug Release Profile of Brand 4

S. No.	Time in mins	Absorbance in nm	Concentration (c) µg/mL	(c × 0.5) µg/mL	(c × 30) µg/mL	CDR	% CDR	Log CDR
1	0							
2	15							
3	30							
4	60							
5	90							
6	120							
7	150							
8	180							
9	210							
10	240							
11	300							
12	360							
13	390							
14	420							
15	480							

Table 8 Drug Release Profile of Brand 5

S. No.	Time in mins	Absorbance in nm	Concentration (c) µg/mL	(c × 0.5) µg/mL	(c × 30) µg/mL	CDR	% CDR	Log CDR
1	0							
2	15							
3	30							
4	60							
5	90							
6	120							
7	150							
8	180							
9	210							
10	240							
11	300							
12	360							
13	390							
14	420							
15	480							

Experiment   13

Gel Formulation

Pharmaceutical gels are semisolid systems in which there is interaction (either physical or covalent) between colloidal particles within a liquid vehicle. The vehicle is continuous and interacts with the colloidal particles. The term Gel represents a physical state with properties intermediate b/w those of solids and liquids. A gel is a solid jelly-like material that can have properties ranging from soft and weak to hard and tough.

Gels are defined as a substantially dilute cross-linked system, which exhibits no flow when in the steady-state. By weight, gels are mostly liquid, yet they behave like solids due to a three-dimensional cross-linked network within the liquid. It is the crosslinking within the fluid that gives a gel its structure (hardness) and contributes to the adhesive stick (tack). In this way gels are a dispersion of molecules of a liquid within a solid in which liquid particles are dispersed in the solid medium.

The word gel was coined by 19th-century Scottish chemist Thomas Graham by clipping from gelatin. Gels consist of a solid three-dimensional network that spans the volume of a liquid medium and ensnares it through surface tension effects. This internal network structure may result from physical bonds (physical gels) or chemical bonds (chemical gels), as well as crystallites or other junctions that remain intact within the extending fluid. Virtually any fluid can be used as an extender including water (hydrogels), oil, and air (aerogel). Both by weight and volume, gels are mostly fluid in composition and thus exhibit densities similar to those of their constituent liquids.

Edible jelly is a common example of a hydrogel and has approximately the density of water. Polyionic polymers are polymers with an ionic functional group. The ionic charges prevent the formation of tightly coiled polymer chains. This allows them to contribute more to viscosity in their stretched state, because the stretched-out polymer takes up more space. This is also the reason gel hardens.

A hydrogel is a network of polymer chains that are hydrophilic, sometimes found as a colloidal gel in which water is the dispersion medium. A three-dimensional solid, results from the hydrophilic polymer chains being held together by cross-links. Because of the inherent cross-links, the structural integrity of the hydrogel network does not dissolve from the high concentration of water.

Hydrogels are highly absorbent (they can contain over 90% water) natural or synthetic polymeric networks. Hydrogels also possess a degree of flexibility very similar to natural tissue, due to their significant water content.

Object

Formulate and evaluate diclofenac sodium gel and comparison with marketed formulation.

References

1. Shivhare UD, Jain KB, Mathur VB, Bhusari KP And Roy AA, Formulation development and evaluation of diclofenac sodium gel using water soluble polyacrylamide polymer, Digest Journal of Nanomaterials and Biostructures Vol. 4, No.2, 2009, 285 – 290.
2. Sera UV and Ramana MV, *In vitro* skin absorption and drug release – a comparison of four commercial hydrophilic gel preparations for topical use. The Indian Pharmacist, 73, 2006, 356-36.

Requirements

Chemicals: Diclofenac sodium, polymer, sodium meta bi sulfite, glycerin, propylene glycol, distilled water and marketed voveran gel.

Glassware etc: beaker, glass rod, funnel, pipette, measuring cylinder etc.

Principle

High molecular weights water soluble homopolymer of acrylamide are reported to possess very high viscosity in low concentration, transparency, film forming properties and are useful in formation of gel. Topical gel preparations are intended for skin application or to certain mucosal surfaces for local action or percutaneous penetration of medicament or for their emollient or protective action. Gels are typically formed from a liquid phase that has been thickened with other components. The continuous liquid phase allows free diffusion of molecules through the polymers scaffold and hence release should be equivalent to that from a simple solution. NSAID's are nonsteroidal drugs having excellent anti-inflammatory and analgesic activity but NSAID produces GIT ulceration, liver and kidney trouble especially in case of oral administration. In view, of adverse drug reaction associated with oral formulations, diclofenac sodium is increasingly administered by topical route. Polyacrylamide is used as water soluble or hydrophilic polymers topically in gel drug delivery system. A range of grades based on molecular fractions of these polymer are available, they are typically used at a concentration between 1 to 5% in topical gel formulation. Due to their non-greasy properties, they can provide easily washable film on the skin. Polyacrylamide polymer of high molecular weight do not penetrate the skin and are nontoxic. Human cutaneous tolerance tests performed to evaluate the irritation of 1-5% w/w polyacrylamide indicated that the polymer was well tolerated. Polyacrylamide polymers have the potential to be naturally broken down and biodegradable and do not persist or accumulate in the environment.

Formula

S. No.	Name of Ingredient	Quantity Given (gm)	Quantity Taken (gm)
1	Polymer	5.0	
2	Drug	5.0	
3	Isopropyl alcohol	5.0	
4	Sodium meta bi sulfite	0.1	
5	Glycerin/ propylene glycol	1.0	
6	Distilled Water	upto 100	

Procedure

1. Weigh 3 gm of the drug and dissolve in iso propyl alcohol. Mix.
2. Add glycerine and mix to get solution A.
3. Weigh polymer and transfer to a beaker containing 75 gm of distilled water and 0.1 gm of sodium meta bi sulphite. Stir to get solution B.
4. Mix solution A to B and stir thoroughly and make up to 100 gm with distilled water.
5. Keep overnight to remove entrapped air if any.
6. Store in an air tight container until use.

Evaluation

1. **pH:** The pH of the various gel formulations is determined using digital pH meter.

2. **Spreadability:** It is determined by wooden block and glass slide apparatus. Weights about 20g are added to the pan and the time is noted for upper slide (movable) to separate completely from the fixed slides. Spread ability was then calculated by using the formula: $S = M.L / T$

   Where,

   S = Spread ability

M = Weight tide to upper slide

L = Length of glass slide

T = Time taken to separate the slide completely from each other

3. ***Consistency:*** The measurement of consistency of the prepared gels is done by dropping a cone attached to a holding rod from a fix distance of 10cm in such way that it should fall on the centre of the glass cup filled with the gel. The penetration by the cone is measured from the surface of the gel to the tip of the cone inside the gel. The distance travelled by cone was noted down after 10sec.

4. ***Homogeneity:*** By visual inspection after the gels have set in the container for their appearance and presence of any aggregates.

5. ***Skin irritation:*** Test for irritation can be performed on human volunteers. For each gel, five volunteers were selected and 1.0g of formulated gel was applied on an area of 2 square inch to the back of hand. The volunteers are observed for lesions or irritation.

6. ***Drug content:*** Take 100 mg of developed gel and marketed gel and dissolve in 100mL of phosphate buffer of pH 6.8. Then, shake the volumetric flask containing gel solution for 2hr on mechanical shaker to get complete solubility of drug. Filter and estimate drug content spectrophotometrically with phosphate buffer (pH 6.8) as blank.

7. ***Accelerated stability studies:*** Subject the selected formulations to a stability testing for three months as per ICH norms at a temperature of $40° \pm 2°$. At regular intervals check for change in appearance, pH or drug content by procedure stated earlier.

Observations

Formulation	pH	Spreadability (g.cm/sec)	Consistency (60 sec)	Homogeneity	Skin irritation test	Drug Content
Prepared						
Blank						
Marketed						

Stability Studies

Formulation	Time Pesriod (Months)	Appearance	pH	Drug Content (%)
Prepared	0			
	1			
	2			
	3			

Table *Contd*

Formulation	Time Pesriod (Months)	Appearance	pH	Drug Content (%)
Blank	0			
	1			
	2			
	3			
Marketed	0			
	1			
	2			
	3			

Experiment 14

Microspheres by Solvent Evaporation Method

Microspheres are one of the most important and successful controlled delivery systems. It has been known that spherical particles can be uniformly covered with polymer film and specific surface area of such particles is a main factor to control the drug release. Microencapsulation and microsphere formulation is a technology devoted to entrapping solids, liquids, or gases inside one or more polymeric coatings utilizing either physical or chemical methods.

A microcapsule is a system that contains a well defined core and a well defined envelope while a microsphere is a structure made up of a continuous phase of one or more miscible polymers in which the drug is dispersed at either the macroscopic (particulate) or molecular (dissolution) level. Selection of the polymer and the method to be utilized for the encapsulation of the particle depends on the final application of the product followed by preparation ensuring reproducibility, high microencapsulation efficiency, and preservation of the activity of the encapsulated substance. This is the replication and optimization of the product.

The multi-particulate systems are considered and accepted as a reliable means to deliver the drug to the target site or to maintain the desired concentration at the site of interest. Polymer microspheres can be employed to deliver medication in a rate controlled and sometimes targeted manner. Medication is released from a microsphere by drug leaching from these polymers or by degradation of the polymer matrix. Thus, rate of release of drug from the microspheres depend on the physical and chemical properties of the releasing medium.

Various methodologies have been used for the preparation containing hydrophilic core and hydrophobic coating as a controlled release system. The influence of excipients and formulation factors on the dissolution behavior of the polymeric microspheres is very important. Controlled release systems provide drug release in an amount sufficient to maintain the therapeutic drug level over extended periods of time, with the release profiles predominantly controlled by the special technologies and design of the system itself. The release of the active ingredient is therefore, ideally independent of exterior factors. The use of drugs with high water solubility leads to a slight acceleration of the release due to the contribution of diffusion to the release process.

Microspheres offer many advantages over single tablets as: small particles will distribute well over the stomach and intestine to give more uniform release, reduce the effects due to local conditions as pH, drug can be coated with different coatings, to give the required release profile. In addition, the size of the dosage form and the thickness of the coat may be altered to vary the release profile, Separate active ingredients can be coated individually.

Object

Prepare and evaluate microspheres for the given drug by emulsification solvent evaporation technique.

References

1. Vyas SP, Khar RK, "Targetted and controlled drug delivery, novel carrier system". 1st edition, 2002, CBS publishers and distributors, Daryaganj, New Delhi, page no – 417-418, 428-429.
2. Jain NK, "Controlled drug delivery" 1st edition, CBS publishers, New Delhi, page no – 236-240.

Requirements

Chemicals: Cellulose Acetate, Acetone, Liquid Paraffin, Span- 80, Drug.

Glassware: Beaker, Glass Rod, Measuring Cylinder, Pipette, Funnel.

Principle

Microspheres are small spherical particles, with diameters in the micrometer range (typically 1 μm to 1000 μm (1 mm)). Microspheres are sometimes referred to as microparticles. Microspheres can be manufactured from various natural and synthetic materials. Glass microspheres, polymer microspheres and ceramic microspheres are commercially available. Solid and hollow microspheres vary widely in density and, therefore, are used for different applications. Hollow microspheres are typically used as additives to lower the density of a material. Solid microspheres have numerous applications depending on what material they are constructed of and what size they are.

The microsphere are characteristically free flowing powders consisting of proteins or synthetic polymers, which are biodegradable in nature, and ideally having a particle size less than 200 μm. Solid biodegradable microspheres incorporating a drug dispersed or dissolved throughout particle matrix have the potential for the controlled release of drug. These carriers received much attention not only for prolonged release but also for the targeting of the anticancer drugs to the tumor.

Advantages of Microspheres

- Increased duration of action.
- First pass effect can be avoided.
- Improved protein and peptide drug delivery.
- Less side effects and increased therapeutic effect.
- Reduce toxicity.
- Ability to bind and release high concentration of drugs.
- Patient compliance is good.
- Method of preparation is simple.
- Can be injected into the body using hypodermic needle.

Disadvantages of microspheres

- Removal once injected is difficult.
- Sometimes non-uniformity of drug content may result while preparation.
- Unknown toxicity of beads.

Procedure

1. Weigh the polymer accurately and transfer to clean and dry beaker.
2. Add acetone to it and allow to wet the polymer.
3. When wetting is over, dissolve the polymer thoroughly by stirring to break any lumps.
4. Add required amount of drug to the polymer solution and stir.
5. Take 100 mL of liquid paraffin in a clean and dried 500 ml beaker.
6. Add 1% span 80 to it and stir for uniform distribution.
7. Add the drug-polymer solution to the above solution using a syringe at a rate not more than 10 mL/min.
8. Continue stirring at 400 rpm, until complete evaporation of solvent takes place and microspheres have produced
9. Decant liquid paraffin
10. Filter the microspheres and wash with n-Hexane.
11. Dry the microspheres overnight and evaluate.

Evaluation

The microspheres will be evaluated on following parameters:

1. Percentage yield
2. Shape, size, colour and odour
3. Angle of repose
4. Percentage compressibility index
5. Percentage entrapment
6. Drug release study

1. Percentage yield

Weigh 100 mg of the formulation and calculate the percentage yield using the following formula:

$$\text{Percentage yield} = \frac{\text{Amount of microsphers obtained}}{\text{theoritical amount}} \times 100$$

2. Physical evaluation

Size: By optical microscopy

Shape: By optical microscopy

Colour: visual inspection

Odour: manual inspection

3. Angle of repose

Place the microspheres in a funnel placed on a tripod stand and allow to pass to form a heap of microspheres falling from the funnel. The angle of repose is given by tan θ.

tan θ = Height of heap/ radius of heap.

4. Percentage compressibility index

$$\% \text{ compressibility} = \frac{\text{Tapped density} - \text{Pured density}}{\text{Tapped density}} \times 100$$

5. Percentage entrapment

Microspheres equivalent to 50 mg drug is accurately weighed and triturated using mortar and pestle. Add the powdered microsphere to 50 mL phosphate buffer (pH 6.8). Shake using magnetic stirrer for 4 h. Filter through Whatman filter paper. Take 1 mL of this solution, dilute suitably (if required) and analyse spectrophotometrically using UV-Visible spectrophotometer.

Calculate drug entrapment efficiency using the following equation:

$$\text{Percentage drug entrapment} = \frac{\text{Experimental drug content}}{\text{Theoritical amount of drug}} \times 100$$

6. *In vitro* Release Study

The *in vitro* release studies of microspheres are carried out in a United States Pharmacopoeia (USP) paddle type dissolution test apparatus using 900 mL phosphate buffer (pH 6.8). Stir the dissolution medium at 100 rpm with the temperature maintained at 37C ± 1°C. Add microspheres equivalent to 50 mg of drug to the dissolution medium. At predetermined intervals, withdraw 2 mL of aliquots and replace with an equal volume of fresh dissolution medium. Dilute the aliquots suitably and measure drug content using UV-Vis spectrophotometer.

S. No.	Time in min	Absorbance	Concentration (X) µg/mL	(X × 5) µg/mL	(X × 100) µg/mL	Cumulative amount of drug releasedµg
0	0					
1	30					
2	60					
3	90					
4	120					
5	180					
6	240					
7	300					
8	360					
9	420					
10	480					
11	540					
12	600					

Results

S. No	Parameters	Observations
1	Percentage yield	
2	Physical evaluation	
3	Angle of repose	
4	Percentage compressibility index	
5	Percentage drug entrapment	
6	*In- vitro* drug release study	

Alginate Beads

Sodium alginate is an inexpensive, nontoxic complex polysaccharide extracted from kelp; whose composition varies on basis of proportions of its monomeric units namely mannuronic acid and guluronic acid. It is a water-soluble and water swellable polymer, which can swell in contact with aqueous environment by many times of its original size and hence used as thickening and gelling agent. The monomers as well as linear polymers affect the physicochemical properties of the formations, structure and morphology of the microspheres. Sodium alginate is a natural polysaccharide extracted form marine brown algae and produces hydrophilic matrix microspheres. These inter-chain associations can be either temporary or permanent depending on the concentration of calcium in the system. With low levels of calcium, temporary associations are obtained, giving rise to highly viscous, thixotropic solutions. At higher calcium levels, precipitation or gelation results from permanent associations of the chains.

Alginate is a linear co-polymer composed of two monomeric units. D-mannuronic acid and L-guluronic acid. These monomers occur in the alginate molecule as regions made up exclusively of one unit or the other, referred to as M-blocks or G-blocks, or as regions in which the monomers approximate an alternating sequence. The calcium reactivity of alginates is a consequence of the particular molecular geometries of each of these regions. Sodium alginate is capable of forming rigid gels by the action of calcium ion or multivalent cations. Additionally, it also reduces interfacial tension between an oil and water phase and is efficient for preparation of emulsion.

When calcium ions are added to a sodium alginate solution, alignment of the G-blocks occurs; and the calcium ions are bound between the two chains like eggs in an egg box. Thus, the calcium reactivity of algins is the result of calcium-induced dimeric association of the G-block regions. Depending on the amount of calcium present in the system, these inter-chain associations can be either temporary or permanent. With low levels of calcium, temporary associations are obtained, giving rise to highly viscous, thixotropic solutions. At higher calcium levels, precipitation or gelation results from permanent associations of the chains. When a drug is incorporated in a hydrophilic matrix, it swells upon ingestion and the gel layer forms on the surface. This gel layer fills the interstices. The release of cationic drugs is more retarded than anionic drugs, which could be due to the electrostatic interaction between the negative charge of the ionized carboxyl group in alginate chain and positive charge of the cationic drug.

Object

Prepare, evaluate and compare sodium alginate beads.

Reference

1. "Vyas and Dixit"; Pharmaceutical biotechnology; Publishers and distributors; Darya ganj New Delhi, Edition-I; Page. no.: 112-113.

Requirements

Chemicals: Sodium alginate, distill water, drug, calcium chloride dihydrate, ferric chloride, barium chloride.

Glassware: Beaker, conical flask, glass rod, filter paper, funnel.

Principle

Various gel forming polymers may be employed for the controlled release of drug by entrapment. The drug is mixed with gel forming material. The resulting suspension is dispersed in an inert hydrophobic phase and gelatin is produced. Subsequently, a washing medium compatible with the biocatalyst is added and formed beads with drug entrapped are allowed to sediment under gravity or gentle centrifugation in to an aqueous phase. The hydrophobic phase and most of washing medium is separated and then the beads are washed with the medium until they are free from hydrophobic phase of necessary formed beads are sieved on screen or nylon nets. In a variation gelatin of polymeric system is achieved by addition of multivalent counter ions. The polymer typically used is hydrophilic polyelectrolyte in nature and addition of multivalent counter ion thus forms polysalts, which get precipitated as a solidified mass. Since this mass is distinctively a water swollen structure of controlled morphology hence termed as isotropic gelatin. The most popularly known example is calcium alginate gel which is obtained from gelatin of a sodium alginate solution using calcium chloride bath.

Procedure

Table 1 Formula

S. No.	Ingredient(s)	Quantity given	Quantity taken
1	Paracetamol	100 mg	
2	Sodium alginate	600 mg	
3	Calcium chloride dihydrate	10 gms	

Table 1 Contd...

S. No.	Ingredient(s)	Quantity given	Quantity taken
4	Ferric chloride	10 gms	
5	Barium Chloride	10 gms	
6	Distilled water	qs	

1. Transfer accurately weighed amount of sodium alginate in a glass beaker.
2. Add 6mL of water and allow the polymer to wet- undisturbed.
3. Mix continuously by using mechanical stirrer to get homogeneous mixture / solution.
4. Add drug in gradual amount with continuous stirring to polymer solution.
5. Stir continuously with homogenizer and add the remaining amount of water.
6. Add required amount of calcium chloride dihydrate and make up the volume up to 50mL with distilled water.
7. Fill syringe with drug polymer mixture and drop the drug polymer mixture to the calcium chloride solution with intermittent stirring.
8. The rate of addition of drug polymer mixture should not be more than the rate 10mL/min.
9. After the complete addition allow 15min of gelling time and then filter the beads and air.
10. Repeat the procedure with other gelating agents.

Evaluation

1. **Size analysis:** Measure diameter of dried beads using electronic Vernier calipers.
2. **Morphological analysis:** Evaluate shape, color and odor of formulation.
3. *In-vitro* **evaluation:**
   (a) *Floating properties:* Take a 500 mL beaker and fill with 500mL of simulated gastric fluid (PH1.2) without pepsin. Maintain the temperature at $37 \pm 0.5°C$. To this add 100 mg of beads and evaluate for floating property and percentage of beads floating.
   (b) *In-vitro release study:* *In-vitro* release study is performed in triplicate using USP paddle apparatus at 100rpm and temp. The apparatus is maintained at $37 \pm 0.5°C$ and 900 mL of 0.1 N HCl as dissolution media. Weigh 100 mg of formulation and transfer to the basket. Collect aliquots at regular time intervals and assay spectrophotometrically.

Compare the properties of the beads prepared using different gelating agents and report.

Observations

Table 2 Size Analysis of Formulation

S. No.	Diameter (nm)		
	Calcium chloride beads (F1)	Ferric chloride beads(F2)	Barium chloride beads (F3)
1			
2			
3			
4			
5			
6			
7			
8			
9			
10			
11			
12			
13			
14			
15			
16			
17			
18			
19			
20			

Table 3 Floating Properties

Time (min)	Weight of beads sediment			Weight of beads float		
	F1	F2	F3	F1	F2	F3
0						
10						
15						
20						
30						
45						
60						

Percentage % of floating beads = weight of beads that float/ total weight of beads × 100

Table 4 Drug Release Profile of Beads using Calcium Chloride (F1)

S. No.	Time in mins	Absorbance in nm	Concentration (c) µg/mL	(c x 2) µg/mL	(c x 100) µg/mL	CDR	% CDR	Log CDR
1	0							
2	15							
3	30							
4	60							
5	90							
6	120							
7	150							
8	180							
9	210							
10	240							
11	300							
12	360							
13	390							
14	420							
15	480							

Table 5 Drug Release Profile of Beads using Ferric Chloride (F2)

S. No.	Time in mins	Absorbance in nm	Concentration (c) µg/mL	(c × 2) µg/mL	(c × 100) µg/mL	CDR	% CDR	Log CDR
1	0							
2	15							
3	30							
4	60							
5	90							
6	120							
7	150							
8	180							
9	210							
10	240							
11	300							
12	360							
13	390							
14	420							
15	480							

Table 6 Drug Release Profile of Beads using Barium Chloride (F3)

S. No.	Time in mins	Absorbance in nm	Concentration (c) µg/mL	(c × 2) µg/mL	(c × 100) µg/mL	CDR	% CDR	Log CDR
1	0							
2	15							
3	30							
4	60							
5	90							
6	120							
7	150							
8	180							
9	210							
10	240							
11	300							
12	360							
13	390							
14	420							
15	480							

Transdermal Delivery System (Reservoir Type)

The importance of drug delivery has increased over the past decades, and significant advances have been made in the development of novel technologies. Delivery of drug through the skin to achieve a systemic effect of a drug is commonly known as transdermal drug delivery, and it differs from traditional topical drug delivery. Some major advantages of transdermal drug delivery are a limitation of hepatic first pass metabolism, enhancement of therapeutic efficiency and maintenance of steady plasma level of the drug. All statin drugs have poor aqueous solubility and lead to low oral bioavailability.

The reservoir-based system is one of the most common controlled drug delivery systems to date. In these systems, a drug core is surrounded by a polymer film, and the drug release rate is controlled by the properties of the polymer (e.g., polymer composition and molecular weight), the thickness of the coating, and the physicochemical properties of the enclosed drug, such as solubility, drug particle size, and molecular weight. Reservoir-based systems are most beneficial for one of the following two applications: (1) a mid-/long-term administration of a medication that is localized to a specific region (i.e., organ, body cavity, etc.). This is usually done if the area being targeted is difficult to reach via systemic administration (i.e., eye, ear) and/or the drugs administered are toxic and may require a long-term course of dosing (i.e., cancer treatments). (2) A drug depot for long-term systemic administration. This is generally administered as an intramuscular or subcutaneous injection or implantation.

Polymers used in the drug delivery systems can be classified into the following categories: diffusion controlled (nonbiodegradable), chemically controlled (biodegradable), and externally triggered systems (smart polymers responded to pH, temperature, etc.).

The polymers that are commonly used in diffusion-controlled systems are usually nonbiodegradable. In these systems, because the polymers are not biodegradable, there is usually no initial burst release, and the release kinetics are determined by the thickness and permeability of the polymer, the release area, and the solubility of the drug. Biodegradable polymers find widespread use in the drug delivery industry. There are two types of biodegradable polymers: natural polymers and synthetic polymers.

Object

Prepare and evaluate transdermal drug delivery system (reservoir type)

References

1. Jain, N.K.; "Advance in controlled and novel drug delivery"; CBS publishers & distributors; New Delhi.
2. Chein, W. yie; novel drug delivery system; Marcel & dekker Inc; New York; 1987; 2-3, 149-153, 185-193.

Requirements

Apparatus: Beaker, Measuring cylinder, Glass rod, Glass plate.

Chemicals:

For rate-controlled membrane Chloroform, Ethyl cellulose, Di-Butyl phthalate (DBP), Castor oil.

For hydrogel Carbopol 934, Diclofenac sodium.

Principle

Transdermal drug delivery system is topically administered medicament in the form of patches that deliver drugs for systemic effects at a predetermined and controlled rate. At present, the most common form of delivery of drug is the oral route. While this has the notable advantages of easy administration, it also has significant drawback namely poor bioavailability due to hepatic metabolism and the tendency to produce rapid blood level spikes, leading to a need for high and/or frequent dosing, which can be both cost prohibitive and inconvenient. To overcome these difficulties there is a need for the development of new drug delivery system; which will improve the therapeutic efficacy and safety of drug by more precise, spatial and temporal placement within the body there by reducing both the size and number of doses. New drug delivery system is also essential for the delivery of novel, generally engineered pharmaceuticals to the site of action, without incurring significant immunogenicity or biological inactivation. The stratum corneum develops a thin, tough, relatively impermeable membrane which usually provides the rate limiting step in TDDS. Sweat ducts and hair follicles are also paths for entry, but they are considered rather insignificant. Properties that influence transdermal delivery includes;

- Relcase of the medicaments from the vehicles.

- Penetration through the skin barrier.
- Activation of the pharmacological response.

Basic Component of TDDS

The component of transdermal device includes

1. **Polymer matrix or matrices:** The polymer controls the release of the drug from the device. Possible useful polymers for transdermal devices are

   (a) *Natural polymers:* eg. Cellulose derivative, Zein, Gelatin, Shellac, waxes, proteins, gums and their derivatives, natural rubber, starch etc.

   (b) *Synthetic elastomers:* eg. Polybutadeine, hydrin rubber, polysiloxane, Silicone rubber, nitrile, acrylonitrile, Butyl rubber, neoprene, etc.

   (c) *Synthetic polymers:* eg. Polyvinyl alcohol, Polyvinyl Chloride, Polyamide, Polyurea, etc.

2. **The drug:** For successfully developing a TDDS, the drug should be chosen with great care. The following are some of the desirable properties of a drug for Transdermal delivery.

3. **Permeation enhancers**: These are compounds which promote skin permeability by altering the skin as a barrier to the flux of a desired reentrant. These may conveniently be classified under the following main heading.

   (a) *Solvents:* These compound increase penetration possible by swallowing the polar pathway and /or by Fluidizing Lipids example include water alcohols – methanol and ethanol, alkyl methyl sulfoxide – dimethyl sulfoxide, alkyl homologs pf methyl sulfoxide dimethyl acetamide and dimethyl formamide.

   (b) *Surfactants:* These compounds are proposed to enhance polar pathway transport, especially of hydrophilic drugs. The ability of a surfactant to alter penetration is a function of the polar head group and the hydrocarbon chain length.

   Anionic surfactants: eg. Dioctyl sulphosuccinate, sodium lauryl sulphate, Decodecylmethyl sulphoxide etc.

   Nonionic surfactants: eg. Pluronic F127, pluronic F68 etc.

   Bile salts: eg sodium taurocholate, sodium deoxycholate, sodium tauroglycocholate.

   Binary system: These systems apparently open up the hetero-geneous multi laminate pathway as well as the continuous pathways. eg, Propylene glycol-oleic acid and 1, 4-butane diol – linolic acid.

(c) *Miscellaneous chemicals:* These include urea, a hydrating and keratolytic agent, N, N dimethyl-m-toluamide, calcium thioglycolate; ant cholinergic agents. Some potential permeation enhancers have recently been described but the available data on their effectiveness sparse. These include eucalyptol, di-o-methyl-β-cyclodextrin and soya bean casein.

Other Excipients

(a) *Adhesives:* The fastening of all transdermal devices to the skin has so far been done by using a pressure sensitive adhesive which can be positioned on the face of the device or in the back of the device and extending peripherally. Both adhesive systems should fulfill the following criteria

   (i) Should adhere to the skin aggressively, should be easily removed.

   (ii) Should not leave an un-washable residue on the skin.

   (iii) Should not irritate or sensitize the skin.

The face adhesive system should also fulfill the following criteria.

   (i) Physical and chemical compatibility with the drug, excipients and enhancers.

   (ii) Permeation of drug should not be affected.

   (iii) The delivery of simple or blended permeation enhancers should not be affected.

(b) *Backing membrane:* Backing membrane is flexible and they provide a good to the drug reservoir, prevent drug from leaving the dosage form through the top, and accept printing. It is impermeable substance that protects the product during use on the skin. e.g., metallic plastic laminate, plastic backing with absorbent pad and occlusive base plate, adhesive foam pad.

Types of Transdermal Patches
(Four Major Transdermal System)

1. Single-layer Drug-in-Adhesive
2. Multi-layer Drug-in-Adhesive
3. Drug Reservoir-in-Adhesive
4. Drug matrix-in-Adhesive

Procedure

Formula

S. No	Ingredients	Quantity given	Quantity taken
1	Carbopol 934 P	250 mg	
2	Diclofenac sodium	100 mg	
3	Ethyl cellulose	250 mg	
4	Chloroform	15 mL	
5	Glycerol	2 mL	
6	Castor oil	1 mL	
7	Di Butyl Phthalate	2 mL	
8	Adhesive tape	qs	
9	Aluminum foil	qs	

Phase-1

1. Prepare hydrogel of carbopol containing diclofenac sodium.
2. Then prepare the control release membrane of Ethyl cellulose.
3. Add chloroform and glycerol in the required amount.
4. Prepare the mixture of EC and chloroform with the help of magnetic stirrer.
5. Add 1mL castor oil as a plasticizer.
6. Add 2 mL Di-butyl phthalate.
7. Then pour in to a chamber of glass plate and place in inverted funnel over it and allow the solvent to evaporate overnight.

Phase-2

1. Fabricate TDDS, using an adhesive tape and prepare a backing membrane using aluminium foil.
2. Cut 1cm of control release membrane and stick up.
3. Finally attach to skin to produce response.

Evaluation of Patches

Physical appearance, weight & thickness: Observe immediately after formulation. On achieving the desired characteristic of the film, subject for one month at normal room temperature conditions. This is done to determine the effect of storage condition on the physical nature of prepared films.

Thickness: Measure using electronic venire clippers, with a least count of 0.01 mm. Measure at five different points on the films and take average of five reading.

Percentage flatness: Cut the film into strips, two form either end or one from the center. Measure the length of these strips to the nearest cm without applying any additional pressure. The percent flatness of the strips is selected as the average percent of the length calculated from the 7cm strips.

Tensile strength: It is measured in kg/cm^2 by enacting the weight onto the specified area of film till it breaks. This is done to find out the flexibility/ elasticity of the patch/film may be encountered at the time of transportation and storage.

Folding endurance: The folding endurance is defined as the number of folds required to break any polymeric film. The folds on the patch/film have to be made at the same point, till it breaks. It is measured manually by cutting a strip of patch of uniform size (4 x 3cm) and repeatedly folding at the same place till it breaks.

In vitro drug release studies: The *in-vitro* release of Drug from hydro gel is studied using locally fabricated Franze diffusion type cell. A $1cm^2$ piece of the formulation is placed in the Franz tube and subjected to analysis. Withdraw samples of 0.5mL at a time interval of 0.5 hours and replace with 0.5mL of fresh media solution in order to maintain sink condition. The receptor compartment should contain 30mL of the isotonic buffer (ph-6) solution. Analyze the sample spectrophotometrically for drug content using spectrophotometer.

Table 1

S. No	Time in min	Absorbance	Concentration (X) µg/mL	(X × 5) µg/mL	(X × 100) µg/mL	Cumulative amount of drug released µg
0	0					
1	30					
2	60					
3	90					
4	120					
5	150					
6	180					

Transdermal Delivery System (Matrix Type)

Matrix systems also known as Diffusion controlled systems are very popular for sustained release formulations. The can be divided up into different types of mechanisms by which they prolong drug release, these includes reservoir matrix systems, monolithic matrix systems and osmotic pump systems.

Matrix system are favored because of their simplicity, patient compliance etc., then Traditional Drug Delivery (TDS) which have many drawbacks like repeated administration, fluctuation in blood concentration level etc. Controlled release systems aim to improve the effectiveness of drug therapy. These systems modify several parameters of the drug: the release profile and capacity to cross biological carriers (depending on the size of the particle), biodistribution, clearance, and stability (metabolism), among others. In other words, the pharmacokinetics and the pharmacodynamics of the drug are modified by these formulations. Interactions between the polymer chains, which can be non-covalent (electrostatic and hydrogen bonds) or have covalent bonds (cross-linked polymers), confer stability to these structures.

The integrity and the behaviour of these structures in physiological conditions allow the controlled release of the therapeutic agent. One such mechanism is controlled release by swelling. Hydration of the polymer causes an increase in the volume of the polymeric structure and the resulting increase in pore size allows diffusion of the aqueous medium within the polymeric structure and thus the release of the drug. In the treatment of a pathophysiological process, it is desirable that the drug reaches its site of action at a particular concentration. This therapeutic dose range must be constant over a sufficiently long period of time to alter the process. The action of the drugs is limited by their degradation, interaction with other cells, and inability to penetrate tissues due to their chemical nature. The chemical nature of many types of polymeric drug carriers, available facilitates, the distribution and interaction of drugs with their target tissue. These carriers also protect their drug cargo from degradation and prevent their side effects.

Drugs application to the skin surface circumvent hepatic first-pass metabolism and major fluctuations of plasma levels caused by repeated oral administration of rapidly eliminated drugs. Depending on the properties of the combined ingredients, a dispensing carrier to provide a stable physicochemical environment that protects the active compound(s) from chemical degradation should be designed, that can be a liquid or semi-solid, monophasic or multiphasic.

Object

Prepare and evaluate transdermal drug delivery system (matrix type).

References

1. Jain, N.K., "Advanced in controlled and novel drug delivery" CBS publishers & distributors, New Delhi.
2. Chien, W. Yie., Novel Drug Delivery System, Marcel & Dekker Inc., New York, 1987, 2-3, 149-153, 185-193.

Requirements

Apparatus: Beaker, Measuring cylinder, Glass rod, Glass plate.

Chemicals: Diclofenac sodium, Eudragit RL 100, HPMC, poly propylene glycol, carvone, dichloro methane and methanol.

Principle

Transdermal drug delivery system is topically administered medicament in the form of patches that deliver drugs for systemic effects at a predetermined and controlled rate. At present, most common form of delivery of drug is the oral route. While this has the notable advantage of easy administration, it also has significant drawbacks – namely poor bioavailability due to hepatic metabolism (first pass) and the tendency to produce rapid blood level spikes (both high and low), leading to a need for high and/or frequent dosing, which can be both cost prohibitive and inconvenient. To overcome these difficulties there is a need for the development of new drug delivery system; which will improve the therapeutic efficacy and safety of drugs by more precise, spatial and temporal placement with in the body there by reducing both the size and no. of doses. The stratum corneum forms a thin, tough and relatively impermeable membrane which usually provides the rate limiting step in transdermal drug delivery system. Sweat ducts and hair follicles are also paths of entry, but they are considered rather insignificant.

Most patches belong to one of two general types – the reservoir system, and the matrix (or drug-in-adhesive) system. Matrix type are the ones where the active ingredient is dispersed entirely in the adhesive. The protective liner is removed before applying, and the film backing remains when the patch is applied. The excipients are unlike those found in traditional topical products such as ointments, creams, and lotions. The backing layer is made of polyester film, ethylene vinyl alcohol copolymer (EVA), or polyurethane film.

E.g., Climara (estradiol) is a typical patch of the matrix type.

Mechanism

Through a diffusion process, the drug enters the bloodstream directly through the skin. Since there is high concentration on the patch and low concentration in the blood, the drug will keep diffusing into the blood for a long period of time, maintaining the constant concentration of drug in the blood flow.

Advantages

- Multi-day therapy with a single application, rapid notification of medication in the event of emergency, as well as the capacity to terminate drug effects rapidly via patch removal, are all further advantages of this route.

- It provides a controlled release of the medicament.

Disadvantages

- This system has its own limitations in which the drug that require high blood levels cannot be administered and may even cause irritation or sensitization of the skin.

- The adhesives may not adhere well to all types of skin and may be uncomfortable to wear. Along with these limitations the high cost of the product is also a major drawback for the wide acceptance of this product.

Procedure

Formula

S. No.	Ingredients	Quantity given	Quantity taken
1	Diclofenac sodium	250 mg	
2	Eudragit RL 100	300 mg	
3	HPMC E-50	200 mg	
4	Di chloro methane	5 mL	
5	Methanol	7 mL	
6	Propylene glycol	1 mL	
7	Carvone	0.5 mL	

1. Weigh required amount of polymers
2. Transfer to a clean and dried beaker
3. Add 1:1 ratio of dichloromethane and methanol in required quantity and allow to soak for 6 hrs
4. Add carvone and PPG
5. Dissolve drug in about 2 mL of methanol and add to the polymer mixture
6. Stir properly using magnetic stirrer
7. Pour this into the glass moulds, place an inverted funnel and allow the solvent to evaporate overnight followed by vacuum drying.
8. Cut the patch into 1 and 2 cm^2 pieces and store in aluminium foil until use.

Evaluation of Transdermal Patches

Physicochemical Evaluation

Thickness: The thickness of transdermal film is determined by traveling microscope, dial gauge, screw gauge or micrometer at different points of the film.

Uniformity of weight: Weight variation is studied by individually weighing 10 randomly selected patches and calculating the average weight. The individual weight should not deviate significantly from the average weight.

Drug content determination: Dissolve an accurately weighed portion of film (about 100 mg) in 100 mL of suitable solvent in which drug is soluble. Shake continuously for 24 h in shaker incubator. Then sonicate the whole solution. After sonication and subsequent filtration, drug in solution is estimated spectrophotometrically by appropriate dilution.

Content uniformity test: Select 10 patches and content is determined for individual patches. If 9 out of 10 patches have content between 85% to 115% of the specified value and one has content not less than 75% to 125% of the specified value, then transdermal patches pass the test of content uniformity. But if 3 patches have content in the range of 75% to 125%, then additional 20 patches are tested for drug content. If these 20 patches have range from 85% to 115%, then the transdermal patches pass the test.

Moisture content: Weigh the prepared films individually and keep in a desiccator containing calcium chloride at room temperature for 24 h. Weigh the films again after a specified interval until they show a constant weight. The percent moisture content is calculated using following formula.

$$\% \text{ Moisture content} = \frac{\text{Initial weight} - \text{Final weight}}{\text{Final weight}} \times 100\%$$

Moisture uptake: Keep the weighed films in a desiccator at room temperature for 24 h. Then take out and expose to 84% relative humidity using saturated solution of Potassium chloride in a desiccator until a constant weight is achieved. The % moisture uptake is calculated as given below.

$$\% \text{ Moisture content} = \frac{\text{Final weight} - \text{Initial weight}}{\text{Final weight}} \times 100$$

Flatness: A transdermal patch should possess a smooth surface and should not constrict with time. This can be demonstrated with flatness study. For flatness determination, one strip is cut from the center and two from each side of patches. The length of each strip is measured and variation in length is measured by determining percent constriction. Zero percent constriction is equivalent to 100 percent flatness.

$$\% \text{ constriction} = \frac{I_1 - I_2}{I_1} \times 100 \qquad \qquad \dots(1)$$

I_2 = Final length of each strip

I_1 = Initial length of each strip

Folding Endurance: Evaluation of folding endurance involves determining the folding capacity of the films subjected to frequent extreme conditions of folding. Folding endurance is determined by repeatedly folding the film at the same place until it break. The number of times the films could be folded at the same place without breaking is folding endurance value.

Tensile Strength: To determine tensile strength, polymeric films are sandwiched separately by corked linear iron plates. One end of the films is kept fixed with the help of an iron screen and other end is connected to a freely movable thread over a pulley. The weights are added gradually to the pan attached with the hanging end of the thread. A pointer on the thread is used to measure the elongation of the film. The weight just sufficient to break the film is noted. The tensile strength can be calculated using the following equation.

$$\text{Tensile strength} = F/a.b \ (1+L/l) \qquad \qquad \dots(2)$$

F is the force required to break; a is width of film; b is thickness of film; L is length of film; l is elongation of film at break point

Water vapor transmission studies (WVT): For the determination of WVT, weigh one gram of calcium chloride and placed it in previously dried empty vials having equal diameter. Paste the polymer films over the brim with the help of adhesive like silicon adhesive grease and the allow the adhesive to set for 5 minutes. Then, weigh the vials accurately and place in humidity chamber maintained at 68 % RH. Weigh the vials again at 1st day, 2nd day,

3rd day up to 7 consecutive days and an increase in weight is considered as a quantitative measure of moisture transmitted through the patch.

Thumb tack test: The force required to remove thumb from adhesive is a measure of tack.

In vitro release studies: The *in-vitro* release of Drug from formulation is studied using locally fabricated Franze diffusion type cell. A 1cm^2 piece of the formulation is placed in the Franz tube and subjected to analysis. Withdraw samples of 0.5mL at a time interval of 0.5 hours and replace with 0.5mL of fresh media solution in order to maintain sink condition. The receptor compartment should contain 30mL of the isotonic buffer (ph-6) solution. Analyze the sample spectrophotometrically for drug content using spectrophotometer.

Table 1

S. No.	Time in mins	Absorbance in nm	Concentration (X) µg/mL	(X × 0.5) µg/mL	(X × 30) µg/mL	CDR	% CDR	Log CDR
1	0							
2	15							
3	30							
4	60							
5	90							
6	120							
7	150							
8	180							
9	210							
10	240							
11	300							
12	360							
13	390							
14	420							
15	480							

Experiment 18

Muco-adhesive Tablets

Sustained-release and controlled-release drug delivery systems can reduce the undesired fluctuations of drug levels, thus diminishing side effects while improving the therapeutic outcome of the drug. The terms sustained release and controlled release refer to two different types of drug delivery systems, although they are often used interchangeably. Sustained-release dosage forms are systems that prolong the duration of the action by slowing the release of the drug, usually at the cost of delayed onset and its pharmacological action. Controlled-release drug systems are more sophisticated than just simply delaying the release rate and are designed to deliver the drug at specific release rates within a predetermined time period.

Targeted delivery systems are also considered as a controlled delivery system, since they provide spatial control of drug release to a specific site of the body. When intended for a part of the body with high tissue turnover rate, such as intestinal mucosa, a drug linked to a mucoadhesive polymer can increase adhesion to the site and increase bioavailability of a drug that has low residence time.

A new approach has been the use of mucoadhesive systems to increase the residence time of the device within the GI tract.

Bio/muco-adhesive systems are those which bind to the gastric epithelial cell surface or mucin and serve as a potential means of extending the GRT of drug delivery system (DDS) in the stomach, by increasing the intimacy and duration of contact of drug with the biological membrane. The surface epithelial adhesive properties of mucin have been well recognized and applied to the development of GRDDS based on bio/muco-adhesive polymers. The ability to provide adhesion of a drug (or a delivery system) to the GI wall provides a longer residence time in a particular organ site, thereby producing an improved effect in terms of local action or systemic effect.

Binding of polymers to the mucin/epithelial surface can be divided into three broad categories

- Hydration-mediated adhesion.

- Bonding-mediated adhesion.
- Receptor-mediated adhesion.

Object

Prepare and evaluate mucoadhesive tablets

References

1. Derle D, Joshi O, Pawar A, Patel J and Jagadale A, Formulation and evaluation of buccoadhesive bi-layer tablet of propranolol hydrochloride, International Journal of Pharmacy and Pharmaceutical Sciences, 1(1), 2009, 206-212.

2. Parodi B, Russo E, Caviglioli G, Cafaggi S, Bignardi G. Development and characterization of a buccoadhesive dosage form of oxycodone hydrochloride. Drug Development and Industrial Pharmacy, 1996; 22:445-50.

Requirements

Chemicals: Drug, Carbopol 971P, Sodium-alginate (300-400 cps), ethyl cellulose, polyethylene glycol 6000, polyvinyl pyrrolidone K-30, spray dried mannitol

Glassware etc: Beaker, glass rod, funnel, measuring cylinder, mortor pestle

Principle

Buccal delivery of drug provides an alternative to the oral route of drug administration. In recent years, delivery of therapeutic agents through various trans-mucosal routes gained significant attention owing to their pre-systemic metabolism or instability in the acidic environment associated with oral administration. Buccal delivery provides direct entry of drug into the systemic circulation, thus avoiding the hepatic first-pass effect, ensuring ease of administration, and making it possible to terminate delivery when required. Attempts have been made to formulate various buccal mucoadhesive dosage forms, including tablets, films, patches, disks and gels. A suitable buccal drug delivery system should possess good bioadhesive properties, so that it can be retained in the oral cavity for the desired duration and should release the drug in a unidirectional way toward the mucosa, in a controlled and predictable manner, to elicit the required therapeutic response. This unidirectional drug release can be achieved using bi-layer tablet dosage form.

Formula

S. No.	Name of Ingredients	Quantity Given	Quantity Taken
1	Drug		
2	Sodium alginate		
3	Carbopol 971P		
4	PVP K30		
5	Spray dried Mannitol		
6	PEG 6000		
7	Ethyl cellulose		

Procedure

1. Weigh each ingredient separately.
2. Transfer drug, Carbopol, sodium alginate, PVP, Mannitol and PEG 6000 to a polybag and mix for 15 min.
3. Prepare 100 mg compress of this mixture using a single stroke of tablet punching machine.
4. Then, place EC and compress again to get the backing layer.
5. Store the tablets in an air tight container until use.

Evaluation

Precompression parameters

1. % Yield
2. % fines
3. Angle of repose
4. Tapped density
5. Bulk density
6. Compressibility index
7. Hausner ratio

Post compression parameters

1. Diameter of tablet
2. Weight and weight variation of tablet
3. Thickness
4. *Drug content and content uniformity:* Dissolve the tablets in ethanol and filter with Whatman filter paper. Evaporate the filtrate and then dissolve the drug residue in 100 mL phosphate buffer pH 6.8. Take 5 mL of this solution and dilute if required, filter and analyse using UV Double beam spectrophotometer.
5. Friability

6. *In vitro mucoadhesion time:* Adhesion time of formulations is determined using rotating cylinder method (USP type VI apparatus) at 37 ± 0.5°C at 100 rpm using phosphate buffer pH 6.8. Take goat buccal mucosa and adhere to cylinder using cynoacrylate glue. Place this disk on mucosa gently with the finger for 1 minute. The time of disk adhered to mucosa is measured.

7. *Swelling study:* Weigh buccal tablets weighed individually (W1) and place separately in 2% agar gel plates with the core facing the gel surface and incubate at 37 ± 0.1° C. Remove tablet from the petri dish and remove excess surface water carefully using filter paper. Reweigh the swollen tablet (W2), and the swelling index (SI) or percent hydration can be calculated using the following formula

$$\% \text{ of hydration} = (W_2 - W_1) \times 100 / W_2$$ *% of hydration = (W2-W1) X 100 / W2*

Where,

W1- initial weight of tablet

W2- weight of disks at time t

8. *Surface pH study:* Use pH meter to determine the surface pH at room temperature.

9. *Dissolution time:* USP type II rotating paddle method is used to study the drug release from the tablet. Use 600 mL of phosphate buffer saline 6.8 pH and maintain 37 ± 0.5°C, with 50 rpm. Attach the backing layer of buccal tablet to a glass slide with cyanoacrylate adhesive. Place disk at bottom of dissolution vessel. Collect 5 mL samples at predetermined time intervals and replace with fresh medium. Filter samples through Whatman filter paper and analyze after appropriate dilution using UV Double beam spectrophotometer

Table 1 Pre-compression Parameters

Formulation	% Yield	% Fines	Angle of repose	Shape	Color	Size of granules
1						
2						
3						

Table 2 Post-compression Parameters of Tablets

Formulation	Diameter	Weight variation	Thickness (cm)	Drug Content (mg)	Friability	Mucoadhesion time (hrs ± sd)
1						
2						
3						
4						

Table 3 Dissolution Data

S. No.	Time in min	Absorbance	Concentration (X) μg/mL	(X × 5) μg/mL	(X × 900) μg/mL	Cumulative amount of drug released mg
0	0					
1	30					
2	60					
3	90					
4	120					
5	150					
6	180					

Experiment 19

Liposomes

A liposome is a tiny bubble (vesicle), made out of the same material as a cell membrane. Liposomes can be filled with drugs and used to deliver drugs for cancer and other diseases. Liposomes were first described by British haematologist Dr Alec D Bangham FRS in 1961 (published 1964), at the Babraham Institute, in Cambridge. They were discovered when Bangham and R. W. Horne were testing the institute's new electron microscope by adding negative stain to dry phospholipids. The resemblance to the plasmalemma was obvious, and the microscope pictures served as the first real evidence for the cell membrane being a bilayer lipid structure.

The name liposome is derived from two Greek words: 'Lipos' meaning fat and 'Soma' meaning body. Structurally, liposomes are concentric bleeder vesicles in which an aqueous volume is entirely enclosed by a membranous lipid bilayer. Membranes are usually made of phospholipids, which are molecules that have a hydrophilic head group and a hydrophobic tail group. The head is attracted to water, and the tail, which is made of a long hydrocarbon chain, is repelled by water.

In nature, phospholipids are found in stable membranes composed of two layers (a bilayer). In the presence of water, the heads are attracted to water and line up to form a surface facing the water. The tails are repelled by water, and line up to form a surface away from the water. In a cell, one layer of heads faces outside of the cell, attracted to the water in the environment, and another layer of heads faces inside the cell, attracted by the water inside the cell. The hydrocarbon tails of one layer face the hydrocarbon tails of the other layer, and the combined structure forms a bilayer. When membrane phospholipids are disrupted, they can reassemble themselves into tiny spheres, smaller than a normal cell, either as bilayers or monolayers. The bilayer structures are liposomes. The monolayer structures are called micelles.

The lipids in the plasma membrane are chiefly phospholipids like phosphatidylethanolamine and phosphatidylcholine. Phospholipids are amphiphilic with the hydrocarbon tail of the molecule being hydrophobic; its polar head hydrophilic.

As the plasma membrane faces watery solutions on both sides, its phospholipids accommodate this by forming a phospholipid bilayer with the hydrophobic tails facing each other. Liposomes can be composed of naturally-derived phospholipids with mixed lipid chains (like egg phosphatidylethanolamine), or of pure surfactant components like DOPE (dioleoyl phosphatidyl ethanolamine). Liposomes, usually but not by definition, contain a core of aqueous solution; lipid spheres that contain no aqueous material are called micelles, however, reverse micelles can be made to encompass an aqueous environment.

Object

Prepare and characterize Paracetamol loaded liposomes.

References

1. Lachman Leon Kanig L. Joseph "Theory and practice of industrial pharmacy" third edition, published by Varghese publishing house, Hind Rajasthan building Dadar, pg 100-115, 430, 761.

2. Martin's Physical Pharmacy and pharmaceutical sciences, 6th edition, Lippinot and Williams, 2010: 17, 563.

Requirements

Chemicals: Paracetamol, Soya lecithin, Cholesterol, Chloroform

Glassware: Round bottom flask, Pipette, Beaker, Measuring cylinder, Glass rod.

Formula

S. No.	Ingredients	Quantity
1.	Paracetamol	20 mg
2.	Soya lecithin	70 mg
3.	Cholesterol	30 mg
4.	Chloroform	1.5 mL
5.	Distilled water	10 mL

Principle

A liposome is an artificially-prepared spherical vesicle composed of a lamellar phase lipid bilayer. The liposome can be used as a vehicle for administration of nutrients and pharmaceutical drugs. Liposomes can be prepared by disrupting biological membranes (such as by sonication). Liposomes are often composed of phosphatidylcholine-enriched phospholipids and may also contain mixed lipid chains with surfactant properties such as egg phosphatidylethanolamine. A liposome design may employ surface ligands for attaching to unhealthy tissue. The major types of liposomes are the multilamellar vesicle (MLV), the small unilamellar liposome vesicle (SUV), the large unilamellar vesicle (LUV), and the cochleate vesicle. A liposome encapsulates a region of aqueous solution inside a hydrophobic membrane;   dissolved hydrophilic solutes cannot readily pass through the lipids. Hydrophobic chemicals can be dissolved into the membrane, and in this way, liposome can carry both hydrophobic molecules and hydrophilic molecules. To deliver the molecules to sites of action, the lipid bilayer can fuse with other bilayers such as the cell membrane, thus delivering the liposome contents. By making liposomes in a solution of DNA or drugs (which would normally be unable to diffuse through the membrane) they can be (indiscriminately) delivered past the lipid bilayer. A liposome does not necessarily have lipophobic contents, such as water, although it usually does.

Liposomes are used as models for artificial cells. Liposomes can also be designed to deliver drugs in other ways. Liposomes that contain low (or high) pH can be constructed such that dissolved aqueous drugs will be charged in solution (i.e., the pH is outside the drug's pI range). As the pH naturally neutralizes within the liposome (protons can pass through some membranes), the drug will also be neutralized, allowing it to freely pass through a membrane. These liposomes work to deliver drug by diffusion rather than by direct cell fusion.

Procedure

1. Weigh and measure each ingredient separately.
2. Take a completely clean and dried round bottom flask.
3. Add soya lecithin, cholesterol and drug to the RBF and dissolve in small amount of chloroform.
4. Continue shaking till a thin film is produced.
5. After film formation, keep the round bottom flask at room temperature for film drying and complete evaporation of solvent.
6. Ensure complete removal of solvent and then add water for hydration.
7. Allow the hydrated vesicles to swell.
8. Store the vesicles in an air tight container until use.

Evaluation

1. Morphological characterization: Observe the formulated liposomes using optical microscope and determine shape and vesicle size using micrometre slide.
2. Zeta potential

3. *In vitro* drug release
4. Stability studies

Observation table

1. Shape
2. Vesicles size

S. No.	No. of division	S. No.	No. of division	S. No.	No. of division	S. No.	No. of division	S. No.	No. of division
1.		21.		41.		61.		81.	
2.		22.		42.		62.		82.	
3.		23.		43.		63.		83.	
4.		24.		44.		64.		84.	
5.		25.		45.		65.		85.	
6.		26.		46.		66.		86.	
7.		27.		47.		67.		87.	
8.		28.		48.		68.		88.	
9.		29.		49.		69.		89.	
10.		30.		50.		70.		90.	
11.		31.		51.		71.		91.	
12.		32.		52.		72.		92.	
13.		33.		53.		73.		93.	
14.		34.		54.		74.		94.	
15.		35.		55.		75.		95.	
16.		36.		56.		76.		96.	
17.		37.		57.		77.		97.	
18.		38.		58.		78.		98.	
19.		39.		59.		79.		99.	
20.		40.		60.		80.		100.	

S. No.	No. of division (x)	Frequency (n)	Diameter (d) x.LC	nd
1.				
2.				
3.				
4.				
5.				
6.				
7.				
8				

Experiment 20

Niosomes

Niosomes are non-ionic surfactant vesicles obtained on hydration of synthetic nonionic surfactants, with or without incorporation of cholesterol or their lipids. They are vesicular systems similar to liposomes that can be used as carriers of amphiphilic and lipophilic drugs. Niosome are promising vehicle for drug delivery and being non-ionic; and Niosomes are biodegradable, biocompatible nonimmunogenic and exhibit flexibility in their structural characterization. Niosomes have been widely evaluated for controlled release and targeted delivery for the treatment of cancer, viral infections and other microbial diseases. Niosomes can entrap both hydrophilic and lipophilic drugs and can prolong the circulation of the entrapped drug in body. Encapsulation of drug in vesicular system can be predicted to prolong the existence of drug in the systemic circulation and enhance penetration into target tissue, perhaps reduce toxicity if selective uptake can be achieved.

A niosome is a non-ionic surfactant-based liposome. Niosomes are formed mostly by cholesterol incorporation as an excipient. Niosomes are structurally similar to liposomes in having a bilayer, however, the materials used to prepare niosomes make them more stable and thus niosomes offer many more advantages over liposomes. The sizes of niosomes are microscopic and lie in nanometric scale from 10nm-100nm. A typical niosome vesicle would consist of a vesicle forming amphiphile i.e. a non-ionic surfactant such as Span-60, which is usually stabilized by the addition of cholesterol and a small amount of anionic surfactant such as dicetyl phosphate, which also helps in stabilizing the vesicle.

Paul Ehrlich, in 1909, initiated the development for targeted delivery when he envisaged a drug delivery mechanism that would target directly to diseased cell. In noisome, the vesicles forming amphiphile is a non-ionic surfactant such as Span-60 which is usually stabilized by addition of cholesterol and small amount of anionic surfactant such as dicetyl phosphate. The first report of non-ionic surfactant vesicles came from the cosmetic applications devised by L'Oreal. The concept of incorporating the drug into noisome for a better targeting of the drug at appropriate tissue destination is widely accepted by researchers and academicians. Various types of drug deliveries can be possible using niosomes like targeting, ophthalmic, topical, parental, etc. Disadvantages of niosomes include-physical instability, aggregation, fusion, leaking of entrapped drug, hydrolysis of encapsulated drugs which limiting the shelf life of the dispersion. Advantages of niosomes include- the structure of the niosome offers place to accommodate hydrophilic, lipophilic as well as amphiphilic drug moieties, they can be used for a variety of drugs, characteristics such as size, lamellarity etc. of the vesicle can be varied depending on the requirement, vesicles can act as a depot to release the drug slowly and offer a controlled release.

Object

Prepare and characterize niosomes.

References

1. Martin's Physical Pharmacy and pharmaceutical sciences, 6th edition, Lippinot and Williams, 2010: 17, 594.

Requirements

Chemicals: Paracetamol, Span 60, Cholesterol, Diethyl ether

Glassware: Round bottom flask, Pipette, Beaker, Measuring cylinder, Glass rod

Formula

S. No.	Ingredients	Quantity
1.	Paracetamol	20 mg
2.	Span 60	50 mg
3.	Cholesterol	25 mg
4.	Diethyl ether	2.0 mL
5.	Distilled water	10 mL

Principle

A Niosome is a non-ionic surfactant-based vesicle (biology and chemistry). Niosomes are formed mostly by non-ionic surfactant and cholesterol incorporation as an excipient. Other excipients can also be used. Niosomes have more penetrating capability than the previous preparations of emulsions. They are structurally similar to liposomes in having a bilayer, however, the materials used to prepare niosomes make them more stable and thus niosomes offer many more advantages over liposomes. Niosomes are lamellar structures that are microscopic in size. They constitute of non-ionic surfactant of the alkyl or dialkyl polyglycerol ether class and cholesterol with subsequent hydration in aqueous media. The surfactant molecules tend to orient themselves in such a way that the hydrophilic ends of the non-ionic surfactant point outwards, while the hydrophobic ends face each other to form the bilayer. Niosomes can be prepared by various methods, including:

- Ether injection method (EIM)
- Hand shaking method (HSM)
- Reverse phase evaporation method (REV)
- Trans membrane pH gradient
- The "Bubble" method
- Microfluidization method
- Formation of niosomes from proniosomes (Proniosome technology (PT))
- Thin-film hydration method (TFH)
- Heating method (HM)
- Freeze and thaw method (FAT)

Procedure

1. Take a clean and dried round bottom flask.
2. Transfer Span 60, cholesterol and drug and dissolve in small amount of diethyl ether.
3. Continue shaking to get a thin film.
4. Allow the film to dry at room temperature for complete evaporation of solvent.
5. Once the film is completely dried, hydrate using water and allow the hydrated vesicles to swell.
6. Store the vesicles in an air tight container until use.

Evaluation

1. Morphological characterization: Observe the formulated niosomes using optical microscope and determine shape and vesicle size using micrometer slide.
2. Zeta potential
3. *In vitro* drug release
4. Stability studies

S. No.	No. of division	S. No.	No. of division	S. No.	No. of division	S. No.	No. of division	S. No.	No. of division
1.		21.		41.		61.		81.	
2.		22.		42.		62.		82.	
3.		23.		43.		63.		83.	
4.		24.		44.		64.		84.	
5.		25.		45.		65.		85.	
6.		26.		46.		66.		86.	
7.		27.		47.		67.		87.	
8.		28.		48.		68.		88.	
9.		29.		49.		69.		89.	
10.		30.		50.		70.		90.	
11.		31.		51.		71.		91.	
12.		32.		52.		72.		92.	
13.		33.		53.		73.		93.	
14.		34.		54.		74.		94.	
15.		35.		55.		75.		95.	
16.		36.		56.		76.		96.	
17.		37.		57.		77.		97.	
18.		38.		58.		78.		98.	
19.		39.		59.		79.		99.	
20.		40.		60.		80.		100.	

S. No.	No. of division (x)	Frequency (n)	Diameter (d) x.LC	nd
1.				
2.				
3.				
4.				
5.				
6.				
7.				
8				

$\Sigma n = 100$

$\Sigma n\, d = $ Average vesicles size $= \Sigma nd\, /\, \Sigma n$;

Experiment 21

Solid Lipid Nanoparticles

It appears that *Mother Nature* was the first scientist offering nanoscale materials abundantly and they were used by the human beings from time immemorial. Several ancient practices have been developing nanoparticles through the traditional processes, but these were not identified as Nano systems or nanoparticles. Ayurveda, the ancient traditional system of medicine in India, has described several "bhasmas," which have particles with sizes in Nano range and have been used traditionally.

Solid Lipid Nanoparticles (SLNs) are particles made from solid lipids, with a mean diameter in the range from 50 to 1000 nm and described in the mid-1990s. They combine the advantages of other carrier systems, especially regarding lipophilic drug incorporation and parenteral administration. They represent an alternative to polymeric particulate systems and are considered alternative carriers for peptides, proteins, and antigens. For macromolecules with hydrophilic nature, it is not expected to obtain high encapsulation efficiency into the hydrophobic matrix of SLNs. SLNs are relatively recent NPDDS; nevertheless, a recent publication presents an exhaustive list of peptide and protein molecules incorporated in lipid microparticles and nanoparticles, such as peptides (calcitonin, cyclosporine A, insulin, luteinizing hormone-releasing hormone, somatostatin), protein antigens (HB and malaria), and model proteins (bovine serum albumin, lysozyme). However, no results on therapeutic enzyme incorporation in SLNs have been reported so far. SLNs exhibit physical stability, protection of incorporated labile drugs from degradation, controlled release, excellent tolerability, and site-specific targeting. These colloidal systems are made from solid lipids (highly purified triglycerides, complex glyceride mixtures, or waxes) and stabilized by surfactant(s). There is no need for potentially toxic organic solvents for their production, which is important in protein formulation. The solid lipid core of SLNs should increase the chemical stability of the incorporation of macromolecules and protect them from degradation.

Controlled drug release for peptides and protein-loaded SLNs, especially for oral drug delivery (which is not the first choice of administration route for these types of drugs), has been shown. Unlike the flexible vesicular carriers, the lipid nanoparticles are made of solid lipids or a combination of solid and liquid lipids. These are known as Solid Lipid Nanoparticles (SLNs). The drug is incorporated between the voids in the crystal lattice of SLNs.

Object

Formulate and evaluate solid lipid nanoparticles of ciprofloxacin.

References

1. Muhlen, A., Schwarz, C., Mehnert, W., 1998. Solid lipid nanoparticles (SLN) for controlled drug delivery – drug release and release mechanism. Eur. J. Pharm. Biopharm. 45, 149–155

2. Mukherjee, S., Ray, S., Thakur, R.S., 2009. Solid lipid nanoparticles: A modern formulation approach in drug delivery system. Ind.J.Pharm.71,349-358

Requirements

Chemicals: Stearic acid, polyvinyl alcohol, dichloromethane, methanol, tween 80 etc.

Glassware: Beaker, glass rod, pipette, volumetric flask etc.

Apparatus: ultrasonicator, mechanical stirrer etc.

Principle

Solid lipid nanoparticles are a new generation of submicron-sized lipid emulsions where the liquid lipid (oil) has been substituted by a solid lipid. SLNs are particles made from solid Lipid Particles with diameter between approximately 50-1000 nm, which are dispersed in water or aqueous surfactant solution. They are made up of solid hydrophobic core having a monolayer of phospholipid coating. Solid core contains the drug dispersed or dissolved in lipid matrix. They have potential to carry lipophilic or hydrophilic drugs. Solid lipid nanoparticles (SLN) also referred as lipospheres are submicron sized particles in the range of 50-1000 nm, made up of physiological lipids that remain solid at body and room temperature and was first introduced by Muller et al in 1991. SLN offer unique properties such as small size, large surface area, high drug loading and the interaction of phases at the interfaces and are attractive for their potential to improve performance of pharmaceuticals, neutraceuticals and other materials. Controlled drug delivery, enhancement of bioavailability of entrapped drugs via modification of dissolution rate and/or improvement of tissue distribution and targeting of drugs by using SLN have been reported in various application routes: Parenteral (intravenously, intramuscularly or subcutaneously). The formulation of solid lipid nanoparticles has many advantages mainly being controlled and/or targeted drug release, improve stability of pharmaceuticals, high and enhanced drug content (compared to other carriers), feasibility of carrying both lipophilic and hydrophilic drugs. Most lipids incorporated are biodegradable therefore SLN shows excellent biocompatibility. They are easy to scale up and sterilize as they are water-based technology. These formulations are less expensive when compared to polymeric or surfactant-based carrier.

A few properties of SLN lead to following challenges which limits the use of SLN like poor drug loading capacity, drug expulsion after polymeric transition during storage and relatively high-water content of the dispersions, entrapment of water soluble drugs, avoidance of Reticulo Endothelial System (RES), controlled and extended release of drugs.

Three drug incorporation models have been established which are as follows:

- Solid solution model;
- Core-shell model, drug-enriched shell;
- Core-Shell model, drug-enriched core.

Preparation of Solid Lipid Nanoparticles

SLNs are made up of solid lipid, emulsifier and water/solvent. The lipids used may be triglycerides (tri-stearin), partial glycerides (Imwitor), fatty acids (stearic acid, palmitic acid), and steroids (cholesterol) and waxes (cetyl palmitate). Various emulsifiers and their combination (Pluronic F 68, F 127) have been used to stabilize the lipid dispersion. The combination of emulsifiers might prevent particle agglomeration more efficiently.

Methods of Preparation of Solid Lipid Nanoparticles

- High pressure homogenization- by hot homogenization or cold homogenization.
- Ultrasonication/high speed homogenization- by probe ultrasonication or bath ultrasonication.
- Solvent evaporation method.
- Solvent emulsification-diffusion method.
- Supercritical fluid method.
- Microemulsion based method.
- Spray drying method.
- Double emulsion method.
- Precipitation technique.
- Film-ultrasound dispersion.

Applications of Solid Lipid Nanoparticles

- Potential new adjuvant for vaccines.
- In cancer chemotherapy.
- For delivering peptides and proteins.
- For targeted brain drug delivery.
- For parasitic diseases.
- For ultrasonic drug and gene delivery.
- For improved delivery of antiretroviral drugs to the brain.
- To the treatment of malaria.
- Targeted delivery of SLN for the treatment of lung diseases.
- In tuberculosis disease.
- In cosmetic and dermatological preparations.
- For potential agriculture applications.

Procedure

- Dissolve 100 mg of Stearic acid in 5 mL solvent mixture consisting of DCM: MeOH (2 : 3).
- In another beaker dissolve 20 mg of ciprofloxacin in 1 mL aqueous solution containing 0.125% v/v Tween 80.
- Mix both the solutions and sonicate using ultasonicator for 2 min at 60 °C amplitude and 0.5 frequency.
- The primary emulsion is obtained.
- Pour this primary emulsion into 100 mL PVA (0.25%) solution at room temperature (25 °C) and stir for 2 h at 1500 rpm.
- Finally, filter the suspension and store as such for further analysis.

Evaluation of Solid Lipid Nanoparticles

1. *Total Drug Content (TDC):* Total amount of drug in formulation is determined by dissolving 1 mL of suspension in 10 mL of methanol. The amount of ciprofloxacin in each sample is determined spectrophotometrically by measuring the absorbance of the clear supernatant at max of 259 nm. Perform in triplicate. Treat the placebo formulation similar to that of the sample and use as blank for UV absorbance. Calculate the total drug content using the equation;

   $$\text{TDC} = \text{concentration} \times \text{dilution factor} \times \text{volume of formulation}$$

2. *Entrapment efficiency:* The EE is determined by analysing the free drug content in the supernatant obtained after centrifuging the SLN

suspension in high speed centrifuge at 16000 rpm for 30 min at 0°C using Remi cooling centrifuge the EE is calculated as follows:

$$EE = \left\{\frac{\text{Total drug (assay)} - \text{Free drug}}{\text{Total drug}}\right\} \times 100$$

3. ***In-Vitro release studies:*** *In vitro* release studies are performed in pH 6.8 phosphate buffer by dialysis bag method using dialysis membrane having molecular weight of 12000—14000 Da.

Place 5 mL of suspension inside the dialysis bag, tied at both ends and dip in the dissolution medium, which is stirred at 100 rpm using magnetic bead and the temperature at 37_0.2 °C. Withdraw 2 mL of aliquot at pre-set time intervals (0.25, 0.5, 1, 2, 3, 4, 6, 8, 10, 12, 18, 24 h) and replace with equal volume of fresh dissolution medium. Analyse the samples after proper dilution spectrophotometrically at 259 nm. The concentration of drug is calculated using the regression equation of the calibration curve.

4. ***Stability study:*** Pack the dried powder in glass vials sealed with rubber caps and keep under ambient temperature and moisture condition (25 °C and 60% RH) for a period of 1, 2 and 3 months. Every month, the dried powder of the stability samples is re-dispersed in distilled water and the stability of the SLN is evaluated on the basis of measurement of particle size and the EE of the suspension.

Table 1

S. No.	Time in min	Absorbance	Concentration (X) µg/mL	(X × 5) µg/mL	(X × 100) µg/mL	Cumulative amount of drug releasedµg
0	0					
1	30					
2	60					
3	120					
4	180					
5	240					
6	300					
7	360					
8	420					
9	480					
10	540					
11	600					
12	After 24 hrs					

Table 2

Parameters	Fresh sample	During and after stability duration
Total drug content		
Entrapment efficiency		
% *in-vitro* release		

Multiple Emulsions

Multiple emulsions are complex system which consist of both w/o and o/w at the same time. There are potential matrices for the encapsulation of bioactive compounds and for the controlled release compounds w/o/w multiple emulsion are system where small water droplets are entrapped within larger oil droplets and they are disperse continuous water phase because of presence of reservoir phase that can be used to prolong release of active ingredients.

Multiple emulsions are novel carrier systems which are complex and poly dispersed in nature where both w/o and o/w emulsion exists simultaneously in a single system. Lipophilic and hydrophilic surfactants are used for stabilizing these two emulsions respectively. The droplets of the dispersed phase contain even smaller dispersed droplets themselves, therefore also called as "emulsions of emulsions". Each dispersed globule in the double emulsion forms a vesicular structure with single or multiple aqueous compartments separated from the aqueous phase by a layer of oil phase compartments. In multiple emulsion system solute has to transverse from inner miscible phase to outer miscible phase through the middle immiscible organic phase, so it also called as liquid membrane system. The two major types of multiple emulsions are the water-oil-water (w/o/w) and oil-water-oil (o/w/o) double emulsions. The most common multiple emulsions are of W/O/W type, although some specific applications O/W/O emulsions can also be prepared.

Multiple emulsions may find many potential applications in various fields such as chemistry, pharmaceutics, cosmetics, and food. These emulsions have been investigated as controlled-release Drug Delivery Systems (DDS), as 'emulsion liquid membranes' for simultaneous liquid extraction and stripping of metals, organic acids and antibiotics, as microcapsules for the protection and controlled release of functional food ingredients, for the formulation of reduced-calorie food emulsions etc. Other applications include the use of multiple emulsions as intermediate products to the preparation of inorganic particles, lipid nanoparticles, polymeric microspheres, biodegradable microspheres, gel microbeads, and vesicles such as polymerosomes.

Multiple emulsions have significant potential for breakthrough applications in food, agricultural, pharmaceutical, nutraceutical, and cosmetic industries in which they can facilitate the sustained release and transport of active material. They can also improve dissolutions or solubilization of insoluble materials. Due to these properties, multiple emulsions find applications related to protecting sensitive and active molecules such as vitamins C and E from the external phase—a process called antioxidation.

Object

Prepare and evaluate multiple emulsion of water soluble drug.

References

1. Vyas and Khar 'Targeted and control drug delivery" reprint 2008; Published by CBS publication distribution 4596 /1-A Darya gang New Delhi 213.

2. Mehta R.M."Pharmaceutics I" Fourth edition 2007; Vallabh Prakashan Delhi; 258.

Requirements

Chemical: Drug, coconut oil, Span80, Tween80, colouring agent, flavouring agent, water etc.

Apparatus: 100 mL Volumetric Flask 250mL, Beaker Funnel, Weighing Balance, Pipette, Dissolution Apparatus, Viscometer apparatus, IR, UV, Magnetic stirrer.

Principle

Multiple emulsion are often stabilized using a combination of hydrophilic and surfactants. The ratio of these surfactants is important in achieving stable multiple emulsions. The objective of this study was to evaluate the long-term stability of water-in-oil-in-water (w/O/w) multiple emulsion with respect to the concentrations of span 83 and Tween 80 In addition, the effect of surfactant and electrolyte concentration on emulsion bulk rheological properties was investigated. Light microscopy, creaming volume, and rheological properties were used to assess emulsion long-term stability were 20% wt/vol Span 83 in the oil phase and 0.1%wt/vol tween80 in the continuous phase. Higher concentration of Tween 80 had a destructive effect on w/o/w emulsion stability, which correlated with the observation that interfacial film strength at the oil/water interface decreased as the Tween 80 concentration increased. High Span 83 concentrations increased the storage modulus G' (solid like) values and hence enhanced multiple emulsion stability. However, when 30% wt/vol/span 83 was incorporated, the viscosity of the primary w/o emulsion increased considerably, and the emulsion droplets lost their shape. Salt added to the inner aqueous phase exerted an osmotic pressure that caused diffusion of water into the inner aqueous phase and increased W/o/W emulsion viscosity through an increased in the volume fraction of the primary W/O emulsion. This type of viscosity increase imposed a destabilizing effect because of the likelihood of rupture of the inner and multiple droplets.

Multiple water-in-oil-water (W/O/W) emulsion and polymeric nanoparticle formulations containing influenza virus surface antigen hemagglutinin (HA) are thought to be suitable carriers for a vaccine delivery system. The multiple emulsion technique leads to high entrapment of HA, while the solvent evaporation technique encapsulated and adsorbs HA within the nanoparticle. Immune responses of these formulations were investigated in rats and compared with the immune response raised against the conventional vaccine. The responses were detected with the hemagglutinin inhibition (HAI) assay. A single administration of multiple emulsion (F1, F2, F3) and nanoparticle introduction in water-in-oil-in-water (W/O/W) multiple emulsion are emulsion systems water small water droplets are entrapped within larger oil droplets that in turn are dispersed in a continuous water phase. Because of the presence of a reservoir phase inside droplets of another phase that can be used to prolong release of active ingredients, multiple emulsions find many applications in industries such as pharmaceuticals and cosmetics.

Multiple w/o/w emulsions contain both w/o and o/w simple emulsions and requires at least 2 emulsifiers to be present in the system when prepared using the 2-step methods. One that has a low Hydrophile-Lipophile Balance (HLB) value to stabilize the primary W/O emulsion and second that has a high HLB value to stabilize the secondary O/W emulsion. The low HLB surfactant is mainly hydrophobic and is added to the oil phase. The high-HLB surfactant is dominantly hydrophilic and is added to the outer continuous aqueous phase. The concentration ratio of these 2 surfactants is important to obtain stable and high yields of w/o/w emulsions. There are 2 interfaces in a w/o/w multiple emulsion. The primary interface, lying between the inner aqueous phase and the oil phase, contains the low-HLB surfactant. In contrast, both the high-and the low-HLB surfactants are present at the secondary interface (between the multiple droplets and the outer continuous aqueous phase). When the hydrophilic surfactant in the continuous aqueous phase exceeds its critical micelle concentration, the resultant micelles may solublize the hydrophobic surfactant that was originally present in the oil phase and carry it into the outer continuous aqueous phase, resulting in a decrease in the concentration of hydrophobic surfactant in the oil phase. This can eventually lead to rupture of the oil layer and loss of the internal aqueous droplets. To maintain a sufficient amount of the hydrophobic surfactant in the oil phase in order to prevent the oil layer from rupturing, a high concentration of hydrophobic surfactant is preferred. On the other hand, to avoid any potential toxicity associated with surfactants, a minimal concentration of the hydrophobic surfactant is desired in multiple emulsion preparation used pharmaceutically,

Therefore, the optimal concentration of hydrophobic surfactant needs to be determined during formulation development. In this study, w/o/w multiple emulsions containing Span 83 as the low-HLB surfactant and Tween 80 as the high-HLB surfactant were prepared. The stability of these multiple emulsions as functions of Span 83 concentration in the oil phase as well as Tween 80 in the external continuous phase was evaluated.

A unique property of w/o/w multiple emulsions compared to simple w/o emulsions is the diffusion of water through the oil phase because of unbalanced osmotic pressures between the internal and external aqueous phases. The oil layer acts as a membrane separating these 2 aqueous phases. Polar molecule dissolved in either the internal aqueous phase or the external continuous aqueous phase can pass through the oil layer by diffusion because of the concentration gradient. In the case of water this is driven by osmotic pressure. Molecules are often transported via micelles of hydrophobic surfactant present in the oil phase. Water diffusion causes swelling, bursting, or shrinkage of the internal aqueous droplets, affecting the stability of the multiple droplets as well as the release profiles of the active ingredients loaded in the inner dispersed aqueous phase. The volume fraction of the primary emulsion in the multiple emulsion in the multiple emulsion system is changed because of water diffusion. Change in the volume fraction of the primary emulsion in the multiple emulsion system is changed because of water diffusion. Changes in the volume fraction of the primary emulsion alters the rheological properties of multiple emulsions.

As with simple emulsions, the manner in which multiple emulsions flow is one of their most characteristic properties. Therefore, an understanding of the rheological behavior of multiple emulsions is important in formulating, handling, mixing, processing, transporting, and storing such systems. Furthermore, rheological studies can provide useful information on the stability and internal microstructure of multiple emulsions. Although there is a substantial amount of literature published the rheology of simple emulsions, little attentions have been given to multiple emulsions.

In this study, the rheological properties of W/O/W multiple emulsions containing the surfactants Span 83 and Tween 80 were determined. The information gathered here is correlated with the long-term stability of the W/O/W multiple emulsions to help elucidate destabilized mechanisms.

Procedure

Table 1 Formula

S. No.	Ingredients	Quantity Given	Quantity Taken
1.	Coconut oil	10mL	
2.	Tween 80	2mL	
3.	Span 80	0.5	
4.	Water	20mL	

1. Clean all the apparatus and dry properly
2. Weigh accurately drug and mix in water and stir it for 15 min at the 100 rpm.
3. Take Coconut oil and Tween 80, mix and stir on the magnetic Stirrer.
4. Mix the span 80 and stir it for 15 min at the 100 rpm.
5. Mix it in the Coconut oil containing Tween 80 and further stir it for 15 minutes.

Observations

Table 2 Density and Viscosity of Formulation

S. No.	Density	Viscosity
Batch 1		
Batch 2		
Batch 3		

Table 3 Particle Size Evaluation

1. **Particle size determination**

S. No.	Particle Size	S. No.	Particle Size	S. No.	Particle Size
1		18		35	
2		19		36	
3		20		37	
4		21		38	
5		22		39	
6		23		40	
7		24		41	
8		25		42	
9		26		43	
10		27		44	
11		28		45	

Table 3 Contd...

S. No.	Particle Size	S. No.	Particle Size	S. No.	Particle Size
12		29		46	
13		30		47	
14		31		48	
15		32		49	
16		33		50	
17		34			

Table 4 Drug Release Profile of Multiple Emulsion

S. No.	Time in mins	Absorbance in nm	Concentration (X) µg/mL	(X × 2) µg/mL	(X × 100) µg/mL	CDR	% CDR	Log CDR
1	0							
2	15							
3	30							
4	60							
5	90							
6	120							
7	150							
8	180							
9	210							
10	240							
11	300							
12	360							
13	390							
14	420							
15	480							

Experiment 23

Fast Dissolving Tablets

Tablet is still most popular conventional dosage forms existing today because of ease of self-administration, compact in nature, easy to manufacture and it can be deliver in accurate dose. One important drawback of solid dosage forms is the difficulty in swallowing (dysphagia) or chewing in some patients particularly pediatric and geriatric patients. The problem of swallowing is common phenomenon in geriatric patient due to fear of choking, hand tremors, dysphasia and in young individuals due to underdeveloped muscular and nervous systems and in schizophrenic patients which leads to poor patient compliance. Difficulties in swallowing of tablet and capsule are also occur when water is not available, in diarrhea, coughing during the common cold, allergic condition and bronchial infection.

Approximately one-third of the population (mainly pediatric and geriatric) has swallowing difficulties, resulting in poor compliance with oral tablet drug therapy which leads to reduced overall therapy effectiveness. For these reasons, tablets that can rapidly dissolve or disintegrate in the oral cavity have attracted a great deal of attention. Fast dissolving tablets are also known as mouth-dissolving tablets, melt-in mouth tablets, Orodispersible tablets, rapid melts, porous tablets, quick dissolving tablet. Fast dissolving tablets dissolve or disintegrate in the oral cavity without the need of water. Most fast dissolving tablets must include substances to mask the bitter taste of the active ingredient. This masked active ingredient is then swallowed by the patient's saliva along with the soluble. and insoluble excipients. It has been concluded that faster the dissolution, faster the absorption (only the unionized form of drug) and onset of action. Some drugs are absorbed from the oral cavity, pharynx and oesophagus as the saliva passes down into the stomach. Thus, the bioavailability of drug is significantly more than those observed from conventional tablets dosage form. The time for disintegration of fast disintegrating tablets is generally considered to be less than one minute. The fast dissolving solid dosage form turns into a soft paste or liquid form for easy swallowing, and thus it is free of risk of choking. In recent years, a variety of improved methods for delivering drugs have been developed with the aim of improving bioavailability, convenience and patient compliance. Some tablets are designed to dissolve in saliva within a few seconds, and so called true fast-dissolving tablets.

FDDTs, as a novel dosage form, have several characteristics to distinguish them from the more traditional dosage forms. Traditional tablet formulations generally do not require taste masking, because it is assumed that the dosage form will not dissolve until passing the oral cavity. Many oral suspensions, syrups, and chewable tablets simply contain flavors, sugars and other sweeteners to overcome the bitter taste of the drug.

Object

Prepare and evaluate fast dissolving tablets of Diclofenac sodium.

References

1. Lachman Leon Kanig L. Joseph "Theory and practice of industrial pharmacy" third edition, published by Varghese publishing house, Hind Rajasthan building Dadar, pg 68-69, 295-96.

2. Martin's Physical Pharmacy and pharmaceutical sciences, 6th edition, Lippinot and Williams, 2010: 17, 492, 563.

Requirements

Chemicals: Diclofenac sodium, Sodium starch glycolate, Microcrystalline cellulose, Dextrose, Talc, Magnesium stearate.

Glassware: Beaker, Measuring cylinder, Glass rod, Pestle mortar.

Formula

S. No.	Ingredients	Quantity (mg per tablet)
1.	Diclofenac sodium	50
2.	Sodium starch glycolate	25
3.	Microcrystalline cellulose	100 mg
4.	Dextrose	50 mg
5.	Talc	4 mg
6.	Magnesium stearate	6 mg

Principle

The oral route of drug administration is the most convenient and commonly used method of drug delivery. However, this route has certain problems such as unpredictable gastric emptying rate, short gastro-intestinal transit time (8-12 h) and existence of an absorption window in the gastric and upper small intestine for several drugs leading to low and variable oral absorption over shorter period of time. These dosage forms are placed in the mouth, allowed to disperse in the saliva, to produce a suspension which can be easily swallowed by the patient. In addition, patients suffering from dysphagia, motion sickness, repeated emesis and mental disorders prefer these medications because they cannot swallow large quantity of water. Further, drugs exhibiting satisfactory absorption from the oral mucosa or intended for immediate pharmacological action can be advantageously formulated in these dosage forms. Fast dissolving tablets are solid dosage forms containing drugs that disintegrate in the oral cavity within less than one minute leaving an easy-to-swallow residue. These dosage forms are placed in the mouth, allowed to disperse or dissolve in the saliva. They release the drug as soon as they come in contact with the saliva, thus obviating the need for water during administration.

Procedure

1. All the ingredients were weighed and kept separately.
2. Pestle mortar was taken and cleaned.
3. All the ingredients were taken and mixed with pestle mortar.
4. Then the powder mixture was compressed using single punch in a multi station compression machine (mini press II).
5. Prepared tablets were evaluated for different parameters like hardness, weight variation, friability and dispersion time.

Evaluation

1. ***Hardness:*** Hardness of the tablet is determined using Monsanto hardness tester. Pick 3 tablets randomly and determine hardness of tablet and express in kg/cm^2.
2. ***Weight variation:*** Take 20 tablets and note collective weight to determine average weight. Then individual tablet is weighed to check weight variation from average weight of the tablet.
3. ***Friability test:*** Friability of tablets is determined using Roche friabilator. Ten tablets are initially weighed and transferred into friabilator. The friabilator is then operated at 25 rpm for 4 min. up to 100 revolutions. Weigh the tablets weighed again and calculate % friability.
4. ***Dispersion time:*** Take three tablets randomly for dispersion time. Place a tablet in a 100 mL beaker containing water and note the dispersion time.

Observation Table

1. Weight variation:

    Weight of 20 tablets =

S. No.	Weight of tablet (mg)	% weight variation	S. No.	Weight of tablet (mg)	% weight variation
1.					
2.					
3.					
4.					
5.					
6.					
7.					
8.					
9.					
10.					

2. Hardness

S. No.	Hardness (kg/cm^2)	
1.		
2.		
3.		

3. Friability

% friability = before friability – after friability /before friability × 100

Initial weight =

Final weight =

% friability =

4. Dispersion time

S. No.	dispersion time (Sec)	Av. time
1.		
2.		
3.		

Experiment 24

Ocuserts

In developing a drug delivery strategy, issues of absorption, distribution, metabolism, and elimination must be considered. The eye presents unique opportunities and challenges when it comes to the delivery of pharmaceuticals. While absorption by this route is bungling, there are few side effects with convention-al ocular dosage forms.

Ocular drug delivery, involving localized treatment to the eye, presents several challenges based on anatomy and physiology. The cornea has an outer epithelial layer that is about five cells thick, an aqueous layer, and an inner endothelium. Drugs therefore have to cross two lipid layers and an aqueous layer to enter the eye. The epithelium is rate limiting for most drugs; the aqueous region, i.e., the stroma, is rate limiting for very lipophilic drugs. The eye is highly innervated, and patient comfort is of paramount importance in order to achieve good compliance. Two approaches used to increase the residence time of drugs in the eye, and consequently, the amount of drug absorbed, are increasing the viscosity of the solution and the use of an insert or hydrogel contact lenses loaded with drug. Polymers that undergo a phase change from a liquid to a gel in response to temperature, pH, or ionic strength also show promise in this field.

Ocusert, a small intraocular insert, releases pilocarpine to treat glaucoma. This diffusion-controlled reservoir system is effective for 1 week, replacing the need for eyedrops applied 4 times per day. With EVA as the rate-controlling membrane, an initial burst of drug into the eye is seen in the first few hours. The ocular hypotensive effect is fully developed within 2 hours of placement of the insert in the conjunctival sac, and the hypotensive response is maintained throughout the therapy. Vitrasert (Chiron), an intraocular ganciclovir insert for treatment of newly diagnosed cytomegalovirus (CMV) retinitis has been launched recently. The insert contains ganciclovir embedded in a polymer-based system that slowly releases the drug into the eye for up to 8 months. Under research and development, a small intraocular insert delivers 1g/day cidofovir to the vitreous humor for treatment of AIDS-induced CMV retinitis for more than 2 years. Tacrolimus may be administered as a surgical insert contained in a diffusible-walled reservoir sutured to the wall of the sclera to provide a slow-release system for the treatment of ocular disease.

Object

Prepare and evaluate Ocuserts of the given drug.

References

1. Sreenivas SA, Hiremath SP and Godbole AM, Ofloxacin ocular inserts: Design, Formulation and Evaluation, Iranian Journal of Pharmacology & Therapeutics, 5, 2006, 159-162.

2. Lachman Leon Kanig L. Joseph "Theory and practice of industrial pharmacy" third edition, published by Varghese publishing house, Hind Rajasthan building Dadar, 118-129.

Requirements

Chemicals: HPMC, Ethyl cellulose, Dibutyl phthalate, Chloroform, Diclofenac sodium.

Glassware: Pipette, Beaker, Measuring cylinder, Glass rod, Funnel, Petri dish.

Formula

S. No.	Ingredients	Quantity
1.	Dicofenac sodium	50 mg
2.	Ethyl cellulose	150 mg
3.	HPMC	150 mg
4.	Dibutyl phthalate	2 ml
5.	Chloroform	10 ml

Principle

Most ocular treatments like eye drops and suspensions call for the topical administration of ophthalmically active drugs to the tissues around the ocular cavity. These dosage forms are easy to install but suffer from the inherent drawback that the majority of the medication they contain is immediately diluted in the tear film as soon as the eye drop solution is instilled into the *cul-de-sac* and is rapidly drained away from the precorneal cavity by constant tear flow and lacrimo-nasal drainage. Therefore, only a very small fraction of the instilled dose is absorbed by the target tissue. Ocular route of drug delivery is one of the most interesting routes of drug delivery due to unique anatomy, physiology and biochemistry of eye. The main purpose of preparing ocular insert is to increase ocular bioavailability of drug. Ocular inserts maintain the drug concentration within a desired range. Fewer administrations are required so they increase patient compliance. Ocular inserts are defined as preparations with a solid or semisolid consistency, whose size and shape are especially designed for ophthalmic application (i.e., rods or shields). These inserts are placed in the lower fornix and, less frequently, in the upper fornix or on the cornea.

Ophthalmic inserts are defined as sterile preparations, with a solid or a semi solid consistency, whose size & shape are especially designed for ophthalmic application. They are essentially composed of a polymeric support containing drug(s), the latter being incorporated as dispersion or a solution in the polymeric support. The inserts can be used for topical or systemic therapy. The basic objective of controlled drug release is to achieve more effective therapies by eliminating the potential for both under and overdosing. Other advantages are the maintenance of drug concentration within a desired range, fewer administrations, optimal drug use and increased patient compliance.

Procedure

1. Weigh accurately the required quantities of HPMC and ethyl cellulose in a beaker and dissolve in chloroform.
2. Add dibutyl phthalate and drug, and then homogenize.
3. Pour this solution in to petri dish and cover with inverted funnel to allow solvent removal by evaporation.
4. Store prepared ocuserts in an air tight container until used.

Evaluation

1. General characteristics: Inspect colour, odour and shape.
2. Physical appearance: Texture and appearance testing was done by visual inspection.
3. Folding endurance: Checked by repeatedly folding small piece of occusert at same place until it broke.
4. Weight and weight uniformity- Take 5 ocuserts and weigh individually followed by combined weight and determine average weight ± sd.
5. Drug content and drug content uniformity- In a 100 mL volumetric flask, place a preweighed ocusert and allow it to stand overnight. Filter dilute if required and analyse the filtrate by UV spectrophotometer.
6. The *in vitro* release- These studies can be done using biochemical donor-receiver compartment model using semipermeable membrane of transparent cellophane paper. It was tied at one end of the open cylinder, which acted as donor com-partment. Place the ocusert inside the donor com-partment. The semipermeable membrane simulates ocular *in vivo* conditions like corneal epithelial barrier. In order to

simulate the tear volume, place 0.7 mL of water for injection and maintained at the same level throughout the study. Maintain room temperature throughout the study. Keep the entire surface of the membrane in contact with reservoir compartment containing 12 mL of water for injection and stirred continuously using a magnetic stirrer. Withdraw 1.0 mL samples at periodic intervals and re-place with equal volume of medium. Analyse drug content using UV visible spectrophotometer after suitable dilution.

Observation

Result

Occusert was prepared and evaluated for following parameters:

1. General appearance:

    Shape:

    Colour:

    Odour:

2. Physical appearance:

    Texture

3. Folding endurance:

Chewable Tablets

Chewable tablets provide additional advantages like greater absorption and increased patient's compliance. Chewable tablets are a convenient alternative to conventional tablets. They have the great advantage of not requiring water, which means that they can be taken at any time and in any place. When used in combination with other dosage forms, like effervescent tablets, chewable tablets offer additional variety for patients, improving the experience and ensuring better compliance. Our chewable tablets can be made with a 'fizzy' effect which stimulates saliva and makes the experience more enjoyable. Chewable tablets also provide a way of converting poorly soluble APIs into a user-friendly form. For people with dysphagia (difficulty swallowing), chewable tablets are an excellent alternative to conventional tablets. In addition, chewable tablets reduce the risk of drug-induced esophagitis - when a tablet is caught in the esophagus and dissolves while remaining in contact with the sensitive esophagus lining. Chewable tablets can help to avoid this problem.

Benefits of chewable tablets

- Create a more 'user-friendly' experience
- Eliminate need to take water with tablets
- Increase compliance
- Convert poorly soluble APIs into user-friendly form
- Overcome swallowing difficulties
- Reduce risk of esophagitis

The United States Pharmacopeia (USP) recognizes and differentiates between two types of chewable tablets: (1) those that may be chewed for ease of administration, and (2) those that must be chewed or crushed before swallowing to avoid choking and/or to ensure the release of the active ingredient. Adverse events for chewable tablets can include gastrointestinal (GI) obstruction resulting from patients swallowing whole or incompletely chewed tablets, as well as tooth damage and denture breakage resulting from excessive tablet hardness. Critical quality attributes for chewable tablets should include hardness, disintegration, and dissolution, as well as all factors that may influence drug bioavailability and bioequivalence. In addition, careful attention should be given to tablet size, thickness, and friability, as well as taste, which may impact the ability or willingness of a patient to chew the chewable tablet (i.e., a patient may swallow whole, rather than chew, a bad tasting tablet). No single quality characteristic should be considered sufficient to control the performance of a chewable tablet. Instead, the goal should be to develop the proper combination of these attributes to ensure the performance of the chewable tablet for its intended use.

Object

Formulate and evaluate chewable tablets

References

1. Jagdale S, Gattani M, Bhavsar D, Kuchekar B, Chabukswar A, Formulation and evaluation of chewable tablet of levamisole, Int. J. Res. Pharm. Sci. Vol-1, Issue-3, 282-289, 2010.

2. Allen L.V., Popovich G.N., Ansel H.C, Ansel's pharmaceutical dosage forms and drug delivery systems, 8th edition, Lippincott Williams and Wilkins, 2005, pp.240,246.

Requirements

Chemicals: Drug, sodium starch glycolate, lactose, mannitol, magnesium stearate, talc, iso propyl alcohol, sodium saccharin, vanillin

Glassware etc: mortar pestle, beaker, funnel, glass rod, measuring cylinder etc

Principle

Chewable tablets are intended to be chewed in the mouth prior to swallowing and are not intended to be swallowed intact. These tablets provide additional advantages like greater absorption and increased patient's compliance. These are quite useful for paediatric and geriatric patients. The chewable tablets can be prepared by direct compression using directly compressible excipients or can be prepared by wet granulation method. Use of super disintegrate such as sodium starch glycholate, cross carboxy methyl cellulose enhance the disintegration process and aid in the faster release of the drug. If required a suitable channelling agent may added such as microcrystalline cellulose or mannitol. Use of highly water-soluble excipients such as mannitol with its sweet taste and cooling effect affect positively water uptake, dissolution and patient compliance.

Procedure

1. Weigh each ingredient separately and pass through sieve number 22.
2. Transfer each ingredient other than magnesium stearate and talc in to a mortor and unsure thorough mixing.
3. Granulate using isopropyl alcohol to obtain a wet mass and obtain granules using sieve.
4. Dry in hot air oven avoiding charring.
5. Mix 5% of fines, talc and magnesium stearate and punch using tablet punching machine.
6. Store the tablets in an air tight container until use.

Evaluation

Precompression parameters:

1. % Yield
2. % fines
3. Angle of repose
4. Size of granules
5. Shape of granules
6. Color of granules
7. Tapped density
8. Bulk density
9. Compressibility index
10. Hausner ratio

Post compression parameters:

1. Diameter of tablet
2. Weight and weight variation of tablet
3. Thickness
4. Drug content
5. Friability
6. Dissolution time

Table 1 Pre-compression Parameters

Formulation	% Yield	% Fines	Angle of repose	Shape	Color	Size of granules
1						
2						
3						

Table 2 Post-compression Parameters of Tablets

Formulation	Diameter	Weight variation	Thickness (cm)	Drug content (mg)	Friability	Disintegration time (min)
1						
2						
3						

Table 3 Dissolution Data

S. No.	Time in min	Absorbance	Concentration (X) µg/mL	(X × 5) µg/mL	(X × 900) µg/mL	Cumulative amount of drug releasedmg
0	0					
1	30					
2	60					
3	90					
4	120					
5	150					
6	180					

Experiment 26

Nano Suspensions

One of the main problems responsible for the low turnout in the development of new molecular entities as drug formulations is poor solubility and poor permeability of the lead compounds. The increasing frequency of poorly water soluble new chemical entities exhibiting therapeutic activity is of major concern to the pharmaceutical industry. The problem is even more complex for drugs like itraconazole, simvastatin, and carbamazepine which are poorly soluble in both aqueous and nonaqueous media, belonging to BCS class II as classified by biopharmaceutical classification system. Formulation as nanosuspension is an attractive and promising alternative to solve these problems.

Nano suspension consists of the pure poorly water-soluble drug without any matrix material suspended in dispersion. Preparation of nano suspension is simple and applicable to all drugs which are water insoluble. A nano suspension not only solves the problems of poor solubility and bioavailability, but also alters the pharmacokinetics of drug and thus improves drug safety and efficacy. Nano suspensions are colloidal dispersions of nanosized drug particles stabilized by surfactants. They can also be defined as a biphasic system consisting of pure drug particles dispersed in an aqueous vehicle in which the diameter of the suspended particle is less than 1 μm in size. Nano suspensions can be used to enhance the solubility of drugs that are poorly soluble in aqueous as well as lipid media. As a result, the rate of flooding of the active compound increases and the maximum plasma level is reached faster (e.g., oral or intravenous [IV] administration of the nano suspension). This is one of the unique advantages that it has over other approaches for enhancing solubility. It is useful for molecules with poor solubility, poor permeability or both, which poses a significant challenge for the formulators. The reduced particle size renders the possibility of intravenous administration of poorly soluble drugs without blockade of the blood capillaries. The nano suspensions can also be lyophilized or spray dried and the nanoparticles of a nano suspension can also be incorporated in a solid matrix. Apart from this, it has all other advantages of a liquid dosage form over the solid dosage forms.

Nano suspension formulation technology has evolved to meet the needs posed by the numerous water-insoluble drug candidates emerging from high-throughput drug screening programmes that emphasize fit into hydrophobic receptor pockets. The solid state of the nanosuspension confers high weight per volume loading, which is ideal for depot delivery in which administration volume is constrained and high drug levels must be administered. The reduced particle size entails high surface area, thereby increases the dissolution rate to overcome solubility limited bioavailability.

Object

Formulate and evaluate ocular nano suspensions.

References

1. Panchaxari D, Shashidhar K, Vinayak M, Anand G and Anandrao K, Polymeric ocular nanosuspension for controlled release of acyclovir: in vitro release and ocular distribution, Iranian Journal of Pharmaceutical Research, 2009, 8 (2): 79-86.

2. Patravale VB, Abijith A, Date R and Kulkarni RM. Nanosuspensions: a promising drug delivery strategy. Journal of Pharmacy and Pharmacology, 2004, 56: 827-40.

Requirements

Chemicals: poorly water-soluble drug, benzalkonium chloride, Eudragit RS 100, Ethanol, Tween 80, water.

Glassware: Beaker (250 ml), Measuring cylinder, Glass rod, Mortar Pestle, Volumetric flask (100 ml), ultrasonicator, mechanical stirrer, magnetic stirrer.

Principle

Local application of drugs in the forms of drops, colloidal carrier system, gel, etc., to eye is the most popular and well-accepted route of administration for the treatment of various eye disorders. Bioavailability of ophthalmic drug is however very poor due to efficient protective mechanisms of the eye. Blinking, baseline and reflex lachrymation and drainage remove rapidly foreign substances including drugs from the surface of the eye. Moreover, the anatomy, physiology and barrier function of the cornea compromise the rapid absorption of drugs. Frequent instillations of eye drops are necessary to maintain a therapeutic drug level in the tear film or at the site of action. But the frequent use of highly concentrated solutions may induce toxic side effects and cellular damage at the ocular surface. Ocular nano suspensions can be defined as colloidal dispersions of nano-sized drug particles that are produced by a suitable method and stabilized by a suitable stabilizer; these can prove to be a boon for drugs that exhibit poor solubility in lachrymal fluids. The conventional preparations are ill-accepted on account of their short pre-corneal retention time, greasiness, vision-blurring effects, etc. The formulation is aimed to prolonging the retention time of medication on the eye surface and to the improvement of transcorneal penetration as well as solubility of poorly soluble drug.

Formula

S. No.	Ingredients	Quantity given mg	Quantity taken mg
1	Drug	350	
2	Eudragit RS 100	550	
3	Tween 80	0.02	
4	Benzalkonium chloride	0.1	
5	Ethanol	5 ml	
6	Water	50 ml	

Procedure

Nano suspensions were prepared by the quassi-emulsion solvent diffusion technique.

1. Dissolve drug and polymer at room temperature in ethanol (5 mL) and sonicated for 10 minutes.

2. Inject this solution with a syringe into 50 mL water containing Tween 80 (0.02% w/v) and benzalkonium chloride (0.1% w/v), in an ice water bath.

3. Continue mixing by mechanical agitation at 4000rpm for 1 hr.

4. Subject the mixture to ultrasonication for 10 min.

5. Allow to gradual evaporation of solvent to form the matrix type nano particles.

6. Evaporate residues by slow magnetic stirring at room temperature for 8-12 hrs.

Evaluation

1. *Determination of pH:* This is done with the help of a calibrated pH meter.

2. ***Particle size and surface morphology:*** This is determined using optical microscope.

3. ***Drug loading:***

$$\frac{W_{initial\ drug} - W_{free\ drug}}{W_{initial\ drug}} \times 100$$

4. ***In vitro drug release studies:*** This is done using the Dialysis membrane-110 (cut-off: 3500 Da) and modified apparatus. The dissolution medium to be used is freshly prepared 0.14 M phosphate buffer solution (pH 7.4).

   1. Tie the dialysis membrane previously soaked overnight in the dissolution medium to one end of the designed glass cylinder (open at both ends).

   2. Place 5 mL of formulation into this assembly.

   3. Attach the cylinder to a stand and suspend in 50 mL of dissolution medium maintained at 37±1°C so that the membrane just touched the receptor medium surface.

   4. Stir the dissolution medium at 50 rpm using magnetic stirrer.

   5. Collect aliquots, each of 1 mL volume at hourly intervals and replace by an equal volume of the receptor medium.

   6. Analyse the aliquots after suitable dilutions with the receptor medium by UV-Vis spectrophotometry.

   7. To check the eventual limiting effects of the dialysis membrane on drug dissolution, carry out separate experiments in duplicate with a solution of saline, freshly prepared 0.14 M phosphate buffer solution (pH 7.4) in pure drug concentrations present in the nanosuspensions.

Bilayer Tablets

Bilayer tablet is the novel technology for the development of controlled release formulation. Developing a combination of two or more active pharmaceutical ingredients in a single dosage form is known as a bilayer tablet. Now a days the use of bilayered tablets has been increased. Bilayer tablet is more suitable for gradual release of two active ingredients in combination. Bilayered tablet technology helps in separating the two incompatible substances in which one layer is immediately released as loading dose and second layer is controlled/sustained release as maintenance dose. Two incompatible drugs can also be formulated into a bilayer tablet by adding an inert intermediate layer.

These are developed in order to achieve modified release of a drug. In case of conventional dosage forms, there will be a wide range of fluctuations in the drug concentration, which therefore results in unwanted toxicity & low efficiency. It offers advantages as it helps in avoiding chemical incompatibilities between API's by physical separation, suitable for sequential release of two drugs, repetitive dosing is required in conventional dosage forms which can be avoided by bilayer tablet, decreases the dosing frequency. Increases the effectiveness of the drug by restricted action at the targeted location, drug delivery is uniform, lower dose of drug is required compared to conventional dosage forms, preferred & convenient route of administration, chemical & microbial stability is more compared to other oral dosage forms, taste & odour can be masked by coating technique, show highest dose precision & low content variability, easy to swallow etc.

Disadvantages include formulation is difficult for drugs with poor wettability, slow dissolution rate & high absorption in the GIT, cross contamination may occur between the 2 layers, individual layer weight is inaccurate, low yield, insufficient hardness & the layers get separated.

Challenges for preparation of bilayer tablets are many and include the fact that the tablet breaks in to pieces when the two parts of the tablet don't bond totally. The two granulations should adhere properly when compressed into a bilayer tablet. At the point when the granulation of the main layer blends with the granulation of the second layer or vice versa, cross-contamination happens. Much expensive compared to conventional dosage forms or single layer dosage forms. The equipment used for formulation of bilayer tablet i.e., tablet press costs high and development of two compatible granulations is must, which implies additional time spent on formulation, analysis & validation. Several techniques are used for bilayer tablets that include En So Trol Technology, Oros® Push Pull Technology, L-Oros Tm Technology and Duros Technology. Bilayer tablet is the beneficial technology when compared to single layered tablet. By this technique even the incompatible drugs can be compressed into a single tablet. Bilayer tablet helps in sequential release of two drugs in which one as the immediate release and the other as the controlled release.

Object

Formulate and evaluate bilayered tablets.

References

1. Naeem MA, Mahmood A, Khan SA and Shahiq Z, Development and Evaluation of Controlled-Release Bilayer Tablets Containing Microencapsulated Tramadol and Acetaminophen, Tropical Journal of Pharmaceutical Research August 2010; 9 (4): 347-354.

2. Rowe RC, Sheskey RJ, Weller PJ. Handbook of Pharmaceutical Excipients. 4th edn, 2003; p 237.

Requirements

Chemicals: Tramadol hydrochloride, acetaminophen, methanol, ethyl cellulose (22cP) s, cyclohexane and n-hexane

Glassware etc.: Beaker, conical flask, glass rod, funnel, mortor pestle, pipette, measuring cylinder etc.

Principle

Acetaminophen (AAP) is an odourless, slightly bitter, white crystalline powder. It is soluble in organic solvents such as methanol and ethanol but slightly soluble in water and ether. It is an analgesic and antipyretic drug that is used for the relief of fever, headache, and other moderate aches and pains. Tramadol hydrochloride (TmH) is a centrally acting analgesic having both opioid and nonopioid effects. TmH acts as opiate agonists, through selective binding to the μ-opioid receptor, and weak inhibition of norepinephrine and serotonin uptake. Ethyl cellulose (EC), an ethyl ether of cellulose, is a long chain polymer of anhydro-glucose units joined together by acetal linkages. Ethyl cellulose is an inert hydrophobic polymer and is essentially odourless, tasteless, colourless, non-toxic, biocompatible and soluble in a wide range of organic solvents. The conventional solid dosage combination is available, and the patient needs to take these tablets 3 – 4 times a day. A controlled-released combination may increase patient compliance by decreasing the frequency of administration.

Procedure:

1. Dissolve Ethyl cellulose (EC, 1 g) in cyclohexane (50 mL) by heating the mixture to 80°C and then disperse TmH (1 g) was dispersed in it using a magnetic stirrer at 700 rpm.

2. Induce phase separation through rapid temperature reduction by transferring the flask containing the mixture to an ice-bath with continuous stirring.

3. Wash the microparticles with distilled water (20 mL) and then with n-hexane (20 mL) and dry at 40°C in an oven.

4. Store the dried microparticles in an air-tight, amber-coloured glass container.

5. Prepare microparticles of AAP (EC: AAP ratio, 1:1) similarly and store.

6. Take 100 mg and 500 mg equivalent of TmH and AAP by direct compression after blending with 0.75% each of talc and magnesium stearate.

7. Proceed for double compression to ensure sufficient hardness.

Evaluation

Evaluation of microparticles

1. ***Morphological studies:*** This is carried out using optical microscope. Size, size distribution and surface properties should be determined.

2. ***Flow properties:*** Determine using funnel method the angle of repose.

3. ***Drug loading:***

   (a) ***For TmH:*** dissolve 41.5 mg of microparticles in 8 mL of methanol to remove EC coating. Add 20 mL of distilled water and make up the volume to 100mL. Take aliquot after suitable dilution and determine drug content by UV spectrophotometer at 270 nm.

   (b) ***For AAP:*** follow the same procedure as above but analyse by UV spectrophotometer at 245 nm.

Evaluation of bilayer tablets

1. ***Weight and weight variation:*** Take individual weights of 20 tablets and determine average weight and ± SD.

2. ***Thickness and diameter:*** Determine using calibrated Vernier callipers.

3. ***Hardness:*** Use Monsanto hardness tester to determine the average thickness

4. ***Friability:*** Use friabilator to determine % friability

5. ***In vitro dissolution studies:*** This is carried out using USP dissolution apparatus II using buffer change method. Use 900 mL of 0.1 N HCl to 2 hrs, followed by phosphate buffer 6.8 for up to 8 hrs to mimic gastrointestinal conditions. Maintain temperature at $37° \pm 0.5°C$ with stirring at 75 rpm. Collect 5 mL of aliquots at regular intervals and analyse using UV spectrophotometer at 270 and 245 nm for TmH and AAP respectively.

6. ***Accelerated stability studies:*** Pack the bilayer tablets in air-tight amber glass wide-mouth bottles (100 mL) with 25 -30 tablets in each bottle, and then seal with aluminum foil. Keep the bottles at $40 \pm 2°C/75 \pm 5$ %RH. Take twenty-one tablets (18 for dissolution and 3 for drug assay) for the studies from each bottle at 1, 2 and 3 months and evaluate for stability by determining *in vitro* release profile and drug content. Determine Similarity factor ($f2$) to compare the difference of dissolution profile after regular intervals. According to FDA guidelines, $f2$- values between 50 and 100 ensure equivalence of two sets of dissolution data.

$$f2 = 50 \log \left\{ \left[1 + 1/n \sum_{t=1}^{n} (R\,t - T\,t)\,2 \right] - 0.5 \times 100 \right\} \qquad .....(1)$$

Where,

Rt and Tt represent dissolution values of the reference and test products, respectively.

Table 1 Pre-compression parameters

Formulation	% Yield	% Fines	Angle of repose	Shape	Color	Size of granules
1						
2						
3						

Table 2 Post-compression parameters of tablets

Formulation	Diameter	Weight variation	Thickness (cm)	Drug content (mg)
1				
2				
3				

Table 3 Dissolution data

S. No.	Time in min	Absorbance	Concentration (X) µg/mL	(X × 5) µg/mL	(X × 900) µg/mL	Cumulative amount of drug released mg
0	0					
1	30					
2	60					
3	90					
4	120					
5	150					
6	180					

Experiment 28

Film Forming Polymeric Solutions

The transdermal delivery of drugs as alternative to oral dosage forms has been the subject of research for many decades. Due to the considerable advantages of the transdermal application route for some drugs different dosage forms have been developed for the drug delivery through the skin: polymeric patches and semisolids. Currently, the patches still represent the majority of preparations for this application route, but the semisolids (and among them especially the alcoholic hydrogels) have gained more and more acceptance in recent years. Although the number of transdermally applied drugs is limited the existing dosage forms are quite successfully marketed for various indications (the annual market volume for transdermal patches alone in the United States of America was approximately 3 billion USD in 2004).

Film forming gels are a novel approach in this area that might present an alternative to the conventional dosage forms used on the skin, such as ointments, creams, gels or patches. The polymeric solution is applied to the skin as a liquid and forms an almost invisible film *in situ* by solvent evaporation. Transdermal drug delivery system (TDDS) and dermal drug delivery system can provide some desirable performances over conventional pharmaceutical dosage formulations, such as avoiding gut and hepatic first-pass metabolism, improving drug bioavailability, reducing dose frequency and stabilizing drug delivery profiles. The aim of this experiment was to search for alternatives to the conventional forms in order to reduce skin irritation, improve skin adhesion properties, enhance the drug release and increase the patient acceptability from an aesthetic perspective. Because of their peculiar rheological behavior, polymeric gels are beneficial in terms of ease of preparation, ease of application, adhesion to the application surface and ability to deliver a wide variety of drugs.

Typical semisolid formulations can be manufactured with a fairly simple equipment. They offer a high dosing flexibility, which is an advantage in comparison to the patches, but they lack the dosing accuracy.

The latter results from the fact that a correct dosing of the drug relies on the patient's ability to distribute the fixed amount of formulation on a skin area of appropriate size. The application sites for the semisolids that are required to produce adequate dosing levels are considerable larger than the sizes of the transdermal patches.

Object

Formulate and evaluate film forming polymeric solutions.

References

1. Schroeder IZ, Franke, P, Schaefer, UF and Lehr, C, Development and characterisation of film forming polymeric solutions for skin drug delivery, European Journal of Pharmaceutics and Biopharmaceutics, 65, 2007, 111-121.

2. Eagelstein, WH, Sullivan, TP, Giordano, PA and Miskin BM, Liquid adhesive bandage for the treatment of minor cuts and abrasions, Dermatological Surgeries, 28, 2002, 263-267.

Requirements

Chemicals: Eudragit RL 100 or Poly vinyl alcohol, Ethanol (96%), triethyl citrate, dibutyl phathalate, distilled water and succinic acid.

Glassware etc: Beaker, conical flask, glass rod, funnel, mortor pestle, pipette, measuring cylinder etc.

Principle

Skin is a very important route for the dermal or transdermal delivery of pharmaceutically active compounds. Film forming polymeric solutions are a novel approach in this area that might present an alternative to the conventional dosage forms used on the skin such as ointments, gels or patches. The polymeric solution is applied to the skin as a liquid and it forms an invisible film *in situ* by solvent evaporation. These are much used in surgeries as tissue glue for the thread free incisions. These film forming solutions can be used with or without drug for minor cuts and abrasions. These can be developed by varying type and content of the film forming polymer as well as the nature and content of the plasticizer. These offer various advantages over patches as higher dosage flexibility, higher patient compliance, rub off assistance etc. Various polymers that can be used to formulate film forming solutions involve Eudragit E 100, Eudragit NE 40D, Eudragit S 100, Polyvinyl pyrrolidone, hydroxypropyl cellulose, polyvinyl alcohol and silicon etc.

Formula

S. No.	Name of Ingredients	Quantity Given (%w/w)	Quantity Taken (%w/w)
1	Polymer	10	
2	Plasticizer	2	
3	Ethanol 96%	75	
4	Water	15	
5	Succinic acid	0.9	

Procedure

1. Weigh each ingredient separately.
2. Dissolve the weighed polymer (500 mg) and add 20 mL of the ethanol and stir for 2 hrs to ensure complete dissolution of polymer after covering with
3. After a clear solution is obtained add dibutyl phthalate or triethyl citrate and succinic acid.
4. Stir for another 2 hrs before use.
5. Store the formulations in glass vials sealed tightly with a rubber plug and aluminium foil.

Evaluation

1. *Viscosity:* Determine the viscosity of the polymeric solution using Brookefield viscometer and rank as low (water like), medium (glycerol like) or high (syrup like). This can also be done visually.
2. *Drying time:* This is calculated by applying a thin coat of the solution ($10\mu L/cm^2$) over a glass slide maintained at 35°C or by applying the solution to the inner side of the forearm. After 5 min a clean and dry glass slide is placed on the film without pressure. If no remains of the liquid are visible after removal, film is considered dry. This varies with the viscosity of the solution.
3. *Outward stickiness:* Press a piece of cotton wool on the dry film under low pressure. If cotton fibres are retained then the stickiness is rated high (dense accumulation of fibres on film), medium (thin fibre on the film) or low (occasional or no adherence of fibres).
4. *Cosmetic attractiveness:* Visually inspect the dry films. Transparent films with a low skin fixation offer high attractiveness due to their invisibility.
5. *Film integrity:* Apply the solution on the fore arm and allow it to stay overnight. After 12 hrs inspect the dry film for completeness of film, appearance of cracks or flaking using a magnifying glass.

6. ***Determination of mechanical properties:*** Transfer 15 mL of the polymeric solution in a glass or Teflon mould (6cm x 10 cm) and allow for solvent evaporation for 72 hrs. Cut the dry films into rectangular stripes of 10 mm x 40 mm. Measure

   (a) *Film thickness:* using Vernier callipers or micrometer.

   (b) *Tensile strength:* using tensile strength tester.

7. ***Water vapour permeability:*** Transfer the solution into a Teflon mould (6cm × 10 cm) and allow for solvent evaporation for 72 hrs. Cut the dry films into circular films of 2.0 cm. take 10 mL glass vials and fill with 8 gm of distilled water, cover with circular film samples and seal tightly with an aluminium cap. Place in a desiccator containing a saturated solution of sodium bromide to get 58% relative humidity. Calculate water vapour permeability (WVP) using the formula

$$WVP = W/ A*t$$

Where, w = Weight loss of vials

A = Surface area of film

t = time

Observation

Rating score	1	2	3
Viscosity			
Drying time			
Outward stickiness			
Cosmetic attractiveness			
Integrity on skin (after 18 hrs)			

Bioadhesive Gel

The primary goal of bioadhesive controlled drug delivery is to localize a delivery device within the body to enhance the drug absorption process in a site-specific manner. Bioadhesion is affected by the synergistic action of the biological environment, the properties of the polymeric controlled release device, and the presence of the drug itself. The delivery site and the device design are dictated by the drug's molecular structure and its pharmacological behavior.

The term 'bioadhesion' refers to widely diverse phenomena, which all involve the adherence of materials (natural or synthetic) to biological surfaces. As an interface phenomenon, bioadhesion is similar to conventional adhesion, except for the special characteristics of biological organisms and surfaces. As such, this term covers the adhesive properties of both synthetic components and the natural surfaces (such as cells). Bioadhesion could also refer to the use of bioadhesives to bond two surfaces together, which is relevant in drug delivery, dental and surgical applications. Therefore, the wide interest in bioadhesion research is due to its implications for the development of new biomaterials, therapies and technological products such as biosensors.

Various interactions between two chemically active surfaces (i.e. not inert) facilitate the bioadhesion process. Strong adhesion can occur if the two surfaces are capable of forming either covalent, ionic or metallic bonds. At the same time, weaker forces, such as polar (dipole–dipole), hydrogen bonding or van der Waals interactions (induced dipoles) also aid in bonding the two surfaces. It is assumed that the surface is uniform and that there is only one main type of interaction between the protein and the surface. The strength of protein adsorption depends on the net charge and polarity of the side of the protein available for adsorption and the composition of the substrate surface. The protein and substrate could either be predominantly hydrophobic, positively charged, negatively charged or neutral hydrophilic. The interaction of a neutral hydrophilic side of the protein with a surface having a similar polarity tends to lead to weak adsorption. Ionic interactions between proteins and substrate surfaces will lead to relatively moderate adsorption. The interactions between hydrophobic protein moieties and the substrate lead to strong adsorption. This illustrates schematically the role of surface chemistry in protein adsorption. However, proteins contain complex arrangements of hydrophobic, charged and neutral hydrophilic groups, such that the resulting interactions will be combinations of the cases presented. The interfacial energy is an important determinant of successful bioadhesion. In systems exhibiting bioadhesion, the liquid environment influences the spreading of one material phase over another. While interfacial contact and chemical bonding interactions are needed for the initial stages of bioadhesion, the interpenetration or interdiffusion between the molecules of the two contacting surfaces will maintain the adhesive bond.

Object

Formulate and evaluate bioadhesive chitosan gel.

References

1. Varshosaz J, Jaffari F and karimzadeh S, Development of bioadhesive chitosan gels for topical delivery of lidocaine, Scientica Pharmaceutica, 74, 2006, 209-223.
2. Kushla GP, Zatz JL, Evaluation of a noninvasive method for monitoring percutaeous absorption of lidocaine *in vivo*, Pharmaceutical Researcher, 7, 1990, 1033-1037.

Requirements

Chemicals: chitosan, formalin 37% solution, sodium hydroxide, potassium dihydrogen phosphate, lactic acid, lecithin.

Glassware: Beaker, glass rod, funnel, measuring cylinder, tripod stand, pipette etc.

Principle

Transdermal and topical delivery of drugs provide advantages over conventional oral administration. The benefits of transdermal systems include convenience, improved patient compliance and elimination of hepatic first pass metabolism. Though, most of the drugs are not applicable to this mode of drug administration due to the excellent barrier properties of the skin. Molecules need to permeate through stratum corneum, viable epidermis, papillary dermis and capillary walls to enter the systemic circulation. Various drugs such as Lidocaine may be used on skin. To improve drug permeation through skin, various penetration enhancers such as ethanol, oleic acid, sodium laurate, lecithin, cyclodextrins are used which change the structure of skin or alter the skin barrier function. Chitosan is a biodegradable, biocompatible and bioadhesive polymer and is a naturally occurring polysaccharide and can be used to formulate bioadhesive gels for prolonging the local delivery of drugs.

Formula

S. No.	Name of Ingredients	Quantity Given (%w/w)	Quantity Taken (%w/w)
1	Drug	4	
2	Chitosan	2	
3	Lecithin	1	
4	Dilute lactic acid 2%w/w	qs	

Procedure

1. Weigh each ingredient separately.
2. Dissolve chitosan in dilute lactic acid. Stir for 1 hr to ensure complete mixing.
3. Add drug and continue stirring for another 1 hr.
4. Add lecithin and mix for 30 min.
5. Store the prepared gels in an air tight container until use.

Evaluation

1. *Viscosity:* Determine viscosity of the gels using Brookefield viscometer at room temperature.
2. *Bioadhesion:* Take excised skin of neonate rat. Spread 0.5 gm of chitosan gel on 2.5 × 2.5 cm glass slide and fix this to the tensile tester using a double side adhesive. Bring the gel in contact with the excised skin of the rat under a slight pressure and keep in this position for 1 min.
3. *In vitro release studies:* This can be done using dialysis membrane or through excised rat skin on a Franz diffusion cell. Charge the donor membrane with 0.6 gm of the gel and fill the receptor compartment with 27 mL of PBS 7.4 maintained at 37°±0.5°C. Stir using a magnetic stirrer at 200 rpm. Collect 1 mL of aliquot at regular intervals and replace with an equal volume of fresh media. Filter dilute of required and analyse by UV spectrophotometer method.

Experiment 30

Dissolution Media Selection

The media typically used in dissolution studies include acidic solutions, buffers, surfactants, and surfactants with acid or buffers. Media with bile salts and other relevant physiologically based ingredients, sometimes called biorelevant media, can be used in regulatory tests, but typically are used as research tools or for in vitro–in vivo correlation studies. Surfactants are used in dissolution test methods to improve the solubility or wettability of a drug. Sometimes the decision to use a surfactant is based solely on the fact that it will facilitate drug dissolution and not on any further study. It is thus important to understand scientifically the interaction mechanisms between different types of surfactants and drug molecules as well as interactions with excipients. This understanding should guide the analyst in selecting the most appropriate media for methods that will be used in formulation development and drug product dissolution testing. Surfactants reduce solution and surface interfacial tension by replacing water molecules on the surface.

Surfactant molecules include two distinct components, the head (hydrophilic area) and the tail (hydrophobic area). Surfactants can be classified as anionic (e.g., sodium lauryl sulfate [SLS], also known as sodium dodecyl sulfate [SDS]), cationic (e.g., cetyl trimethyl ammonium bromide [CTAB]), zwitterionic (e.g., alkyl betaine), or nonionic (e.g., Tween or Cremophor EL). In dosage systems that contain polymer, the interactions between polymers and surfactants in aqueous media give rise to the formation of association structures, thereby modifying the solution and interfacial properties. The morphologies of association complexes depend on the molecular properties of the polymer and the surfactant. The presence of a polymer lowers the CMC and reduces the size of spherical micelles.

Dissolution is the process by which a solid substance enters the solvent phase to yield a solution i.e. mass transfer from solid surface to liquid phase" and dissolution rate is the amount of drug substance that goes in solution per unit time under standardized conditions of temperature and solvent composition.

Importance

- Dissolution testing is mainly used to confirm product quality and batch-to-batch consistency.

- Dissolution testing finds application in bioavailability problems and bioequivalence studies.

- In R&D department, comparing *In vitro* dissolution data with *In vivo* bioavailability, we would greatly facilitate product development.

Object

Selection of dissolution media for poorly water-soluble drugs.

References

1. Patil PB, Gupta VRM, Udupi RH, Srikanth K and Prasad BS, Development of dissolution medium for poorly water-soluble drug mefenamic acid, 1(4), 2010, 544-549.

2. USP 23, US Pharmacopoeial convention, Rockville, M.D.,1995,267.

Requirements

Chemicals: Mefenamic acid, sodium lauryl sulphate, Tween 80, magnesium stearate talc, distilled water etc.

Glassware etc: Beaker, glass rod, funnel, measuring cylinder, hard gelatin capsules, pipette etc.

Principle

Mefenamic acid, a non-steroidal anti-inflammatory drug, is a potent nonsteroidal anti-inflammatory drug (NSAID) of the enolic acid class, which shows preferential inhibition of cyclooxygenase- 2(COX -2) and inhibits the prostaglandin synthesis. It is highly prescribed in the treatment of rheumatoid arthritis, osteoarthritis and other joint disorders. However, its oral bioavailability is very low, probably due to poor solubility in water and insufficient dissolution rate. Addition of surfactant to the dissolution medium improves the dissolution of pure drug by facilitating the drug release process at the solid/liquid interface and micelle solubilization in the bulk. Its solubility can be increased using cyclodextrins but they have certain disadvantages. Certain types of cyclodextrins have specific toxicity in pre-clinical models potentially thereby limiting their use in toxic studies. Sometimes, the complexed drug with cyclodextrins will not dissociates rapidly, in such cases, the pharmacokinetics of the poorly soluble drug may be altered as release is not immediate. Drugs that are practically insoluble (solubility less than 0.01%) are of increasing therapeutic interest, as it is a well-recognized fact that when administered orally, they may present serious problems of bio-availability. Since their dissolution rate can be the rate limiting step in the *in vivo* absorption process, there is a definite need for the development of an appropriate dissolution test. Approaches usually used in the design of dissolution media for poorly water-soluble drugs include:

(a) Bringing about drug solubility by increasing the volume of the aqueous sink or removing the dissolved drug.

(b) Solubilization of the drug by co-solvents, up to 40% and by anionic or non-ionic surfactants by adding to the dissolution medium in post micellar concentrations.

(c) Alteration of pH to enhance the solubility of insoluble drug molecules. The last two approaches seen less cumbersome and have been more widely employed in pharmacopoeial dissolution tests.

Table 1 Solubility of Mefenamic acid in different solvents

S. No.	Solvents	Saturation Solubility (µg/mL)
1	Water	4.18
2	pH 1.2	6.21
3	pH 6.8	7.01
4	pH 7.4	8.29
5	pH 8.0	7.42
6	5% v/v Methanol in Water	6.33
7	0.5% v/v Tween 80 in Water	112.04
8	1% v/v Tween 80 in Water	214.78
9	0.5% w/v SLS in water	201.28
10	1% w/v SLS in water	401.11

Formula

S. No.	Name of Ingredient	Quantity Given	Quantity Taken
1	Mefenamic acid	100 mg	
2	Magnesium stearate	0.5% w/w	
3	Talc	0.5% w/w	
4	Hard gelatine capsules	...	

Procedure

1. Weigh mefenamic acid and transfer to mortar.
2. Add 0.5% w/w of magnesium stearate and talc.
3. Mix to get a homogeneous mixture.
4. Transfer to hard gelatine capsule.
5. Make 10 such capsule for each media.

Evaluation

1. Weight and weight variation- Individually weigh 10 capsules and find out the average weight.

2. Solubility studies- Weigh 25 mg Mefenamic acid and add to 25ml of water in a conical flask. Keep the conical flasks on a shaker incubator maintained at 37 ± 0.50c for 48hrs. After shaking, filter the solution through Whatman filter paper and assay the filtrate was spectro-photometrically at 285 nm against the respective blank solutions.

3. Dissolution studies- Perform dissolution studies performed using USP dissolution apparatus II at 37 ± 0.5°C and at 50 rpm. Water and water containing SLS of different concentration used as dissolution medium. Withdraw 5 mL of samples at regular intervals and replace with fresh prewarmed media to maintain sink conditions. Analyse the samples spectrophotometrically at 285nm.

4. Draw graph between time and % cumulative drug released.

Observations

S. No.	Time (min)	Water	0.25 % SLS	0.5% SLS	1.0% SLS	1.5% SLS	2.0 % SLS
1	0						
2	5						
3	10						
4	15						
5	30						
6	45						
7	60						
8	75						
9	90						
10	105						

Experiment 31

In Vitro Rate of Absorption Determination

Although there have been tremendous innovations in different drug delivery systems, the oral route is still the most widespread and popular drug administration method by virtue of its convenience, low cost and high patient compliance compared with alternative routes. However, the vulnerability of many drugs to the harsh conditions of the gastrointestinal (GI) tract and the possibility of chemical and enzymatic degradation results in poor therapeutic efficacy of many orally administered drugs.

In fact, oral administration, like other administration routes, faces major obstacles relating to the effective delivery of therapeutics, with the most severe of these being the possibility of drug degradation, negligible transport of drugs across the intestinal epithelium, decreased efficacy due to pH variations and the presence of digestive enzymes, and cell membrane barriers in the GI tract. Thus, it is important to design appropriate models for predicting and screening the permeability and absorption of nanoparticulate drug delivery systems in the intestine. At present, the intestinal absorption models of oral based drug delivery systems can be classified into three categories comprising a total of eight different measurement methods, namely *in vitro* (dialysis bag, rat gut sac, using chamber, and cell culture model), *in situ* (intestinal perfusion, intestinal loops, and intestinal vascular cannulation) and *in vivo* (the blood/urine drug concentration method).

In vitro methods are simple and convenient to perform. It is easy to control the experimental conditions and environment, and the results are reproducible. However, these methods cannot fully reflect the actual absorption of nanoparticles *in vivo* and are therefore usually used to study intestinal absorption mechanisms.

In situ methods mainly refer to experiments on whole animals, where complete blood supply and nerve domination are present, and most importantly, where the intestinal nerve remains intact. These methods directly reflect drug absorption *in situ* and are therefore commonly used to study drug penetration and absorption kinetics. *In situ* methods include intestinal perfusion, intestinal loops, and intestinal vascular cannulation.

No matter how sophisticated an *in vitro* model is, *in vivo* evaluation will eventually be required to validate the true performance of an oral drug delivery system. Noninvasive monitoring is naturally preferred, but such options and the type of data extracted are inherently limited. Data from one intestinal absorption model alone cannot be considered to provide a conclusive result; therefore, simultaneous utilization of two or more independent models is favored by most researchers when studying intestinal absorption.

Object

Determination of rate of *in-vitro* absorption of the given drug using everted intestinal sac.

References

1. Tipnis HP, Nagarsenkar MS, Introduction to biopharmaceutics and pharmacokinetics, Nirali prakashan, 2003, 8-23.

2. Lieberman HA, Lachman L and Shwartz JB, pharmaceutical dosage forms, tablets, vol 2, 350-385.

3. Rowland M, Tozer TN, Clinical pharmacokinetics, concepts and applications, 3rd edition, 11-17.

Requirements

Chemicals: Sodium di hydrogen phosphate, potassium di hydrogen o phosphate, sodium chloride, calcium chloride etc.

Glassware: Volumetric flasks, funnel, beaker, pipette, measuring cylinder etc.

Apparatus etc.: Aerator assembly, electronic balance, pH meter, UV- Vis spectrophotometer.

Principle

To characterize the GI absorption, everted sac technique is used and it gives information to understand the region from which the absorption is optimum, the mechanism involved and kinetics of drug absorption.

A small segment of intestine is isolated and everted to get a sac which is filled with biological media. Both ends are ligated with catgut and the sac is immersed in Erlenmeyer flask containing a relatively large volume of buffer solution that contain drug. The solution inside is called serosal fluid and drug solution outside is called as mucosal fluid. This is then oxygenated and agitated at 37°C for a specific period of time. After incubation, serosal fluid is analysed for drug content. Due to altered supply of blood in the small intestine, *ex vivo*, the rate of transport of drug across everted sac may be slower than in intact animal.

Procedure

1. Collect chick intestine and preserve in PBS 7.4 in cold condition
2. Flush the lumen with cold water.
3. Evert using smooth glass rod, stretch with a spatula and cut at about 5-15 cm of small intestine.
4. Ligate two segments leaving one end loose to allow a blunt needle to pass through.
5. Fill 2 mL of Kreb's mammalian ringer solution and ligate tightly.
6. Suspend in medium containing known amount of drug (100 mL).
7. After 120 min, remove the sac and analyse the serosal fluid and analyse the serosal fluid by UV to estimate amount of drug absorbed.

Time (min)	Absorbance	Concentration (µg/mL)	Total amount of drug absorbed (µg/mL)
45			
90			
120			

Result

The drug shows absorption rate of .... µg/mL.

In Vitro In Vivo Correlation

Drug absorption is measured *in vivo*, in other words in a human (or animal) body. Typical *in vivo* indicators are 'time – blood plasma concentration profiles' of drugs after oral administration. To identify the parameters involved in drug absorption *in vitro* investigations are usually performed. *In vitro* literally means 'in glass' and depicts an investigation performed in an artificial environment mimicking a biological condition. To establish a reliable *in vitro in vivo* relationship (IVIVC) it is important that the artificial environments simulate the biological conditions as closely as possible. On that basis the experimental results can directly be connected to real outcomes in humans. During drug development and formulation exploration, *in vitro* solubility and dissolution should artificially mimic the *in vivo* drug or formulation performance in the human gastrointestinal tract. The *in vitro* results are then related to *in vivo* drug plasma concentration profiles (see danazol example below). When an *in vitro in vivo* correlation is established, it is used for development and optimisation of drug formulations. Research organisations often use this method to reduce costly and time intensive trials on animals and humans during formulation development.

Nowadays, computer models are often used to link *in vitro* results with *in vivo* outcomes. These so called physiologically based pharma-cokinetic (PBPK) models are capable of translating *in vitro* results into *in vivo* predictions. This method is defined as *in vitro in silico in vivo* correlation (*IVISIVC*). Establishing *in vitro in vivo* correlations for poorly soluble drugs (also referred as BCS Class II and IV) can be challenging. When it comes to investigation of drug dissolution performance in the simulated conditions of the gastrointestinal tract, simple buffers usually are not sufficient enough. In this case, Biorelevant Media should be utilized because they closely mimic the fluids of the human (and animal) stomach and intestine. Biorelevant Media have become the gold standard for *IVIVC* and *IVISIVC* investigations of poorly soluble drugs during formulation development.

In vitro in vivo correlations *(IVIVC)* play a key role in the drug development and optimization of formulation which is certainly a time consuming and expensive process. Formulation optimization requires alteration in formulation, composition, equipment, batch sizes and manufacturing process. If such types of one or more changes are applied to the formulation, the *in vivo* bioequivalence studies in human may require to be done to prove the similarity of the new formulation which will not only increase the burden of carrying out a number of bioequivalence studies but eventually increase the cost of the optimization process and ultimately marketing of the new formulation. To overcome these problems, it is desirable to develop in vitro tests that reflect can bioavailability data. IVIVC can be used in the development of new pharmaceuticals to reduce the number of human studies during the formulation development. Thus, the main objective of an IVIVC is to serve as a surrogate for *in vivo* bioavailability and to support biowaivers. IVIVC is a mathematical relationship between *in vitro* properties of a dosage form with its *in vivo* performance. The *In vitro* release data of a dosage form containing the active substance serve as characteristic *in vitro* property, while the *In vivo* performance is generally represented by the time course of the plasma concentration of the active substance. These *In vitro & In vivo* data are then treated scientifically to determine correlations. For oral dosage forms, the *in vitro* release is usually measured and considered as dissolution rate. The relationship between the *in vitro* and *in vivo* characteristics can be expressed mathematically by a linear or nonlinear correlation. However, the plasma concentration cannot be directly correlated to the *in vitro* release rate; it has to be converted to the *in vivo* release or absorption data, either by pharmacokinetic compartment model analysis or by linear system analysis.

An *In-vitro in-vivo* correlation (IVIVC) has been defined by the Food and Drug Administration (FDA) as "a predictive mathematical model describing the relationship between an *in-vitro* property of a dosage form and an *in-vivo* response". Generally, the *In vitro* property is the rate or extent of drug dissolution or release while the In vivo response is the plasma drug concentration or amount of drug absorbed. Practically, the purpose of IVIVC is to use drug dissolution results from two or more products to predict similarity or dissimilarity of expected plasma drug concentration (profiles). Before one considers relating *in vitro* results to *in vivo*, one has to establish as to how one will establish similarity or dissimilarity of *in vivo* response i.e. plasma drug concentration profiles. The methodology of establishing similarity or dissimilarity of plasma drug concentrations profile is commonly known as bioequivalence testing. There are very well established guidance and standards available for establishing bioequivalence between drug profiles and products.

Object

Establishment of IVIVC for given sample of drug.

References

1. Todd PA, Sorkin EM, Diclofenac sodium: A reappraisal of its pharmacodynamic and pharmacokinetic property, therapy efficacy, drugs, 1968, 244-85.

2. Rowland M, Tozer TN, Clinical pharmacokinetics-concepts and applications, Lea and Febiger, 1995, 137-500.

3. Shargel L, Wu-pong S, Yu A, Applied biopharmacokinetics and pharmacokinetics, 4th edition, Prentice Hall Int, 29-61.

Requirements

Chemicals: Diclofenac sodium pure drug and marketed sample, 0.1 N hydrochloric acid, PBS 7.4, 6.8, methanol etc.

Glass wares: Volumetric flask, pipette, funnel, burette stand etc.

Apparatus etc.: pH meter, UV-Vis spectrophotometer etc.

Principle

Diclofenac sodium belongs to group of medicines called as NSAIDs. It is used in the treatment of pain and inflammation occurring due to various patho-physiological conditions. *In vitro in vivo* correlation (IVIVC) as per USFDA is defined as 'a predicative mathematical model depicting the relationship between an *in vitro* property of a dosage form and an *in vivo* response. *In vitro* is generally, rate of extent of dissolution or release while *in vivo* response is amount of drug absorbed. As per USFDA, there are 4 levels of IVIVC and an addition level D is also studied.

Level A: correlated entire *in vitro* and *in vivo* profiles.

Level B: based on principles of statistical moment analysis and used mean *in vitro* dissolution time to mean residence time.

Level C: relates one dissolution time point ($t_{50\%, 90\%}$ etc) to one mean pharmacokinetic parameter as AUC, t_{max} and C_{max}.

Level D: It is not a formal correlation but a semi quantitative method.

Procedure

1. ***In vivo study***

   (a) To simulate in vivo studies, egg membrane is used as the mucosal membrane of stomach

   (b) Prepare stock solution of drug to get a concentration of 3 mg/mL.

   (c) Take 10 mL of this and transfer to donor over dissolution media.

(d) Maintain temperature and rpm optimum.

(e) Collect aliquots at regular interval, analyse spectrophotometrically.

2. *In vitro study*

(a) Take a tablet of marketed drug preparation and carry out dissolution in PBS. Collect aliquots at regular interval and analyse spectrophotometrically.

3. *Determine IVIVC*

Observation Table

S. No.	Time (min)	Absorbance	Concentration X	X × 5	X × 200	Cum Amount	% Cum Amount
1	0						
2	5						
3	10						
4	15						
5	20						
6	30						
7	40						
8	50						
9	60						
10	90						
11	120						
12	150						
13	210						
14	270						

S. No.	Time (min)	Absorbance	Concentration X	X × 5	X × 200	Cum Amount	% Cum Amount
1	0						
2	15						
3	30						
4	45						
5	60						
6	90						
7	120						
8	135						
9	150						
10	180						
11	210						
12	270						

In vitro Dissolution

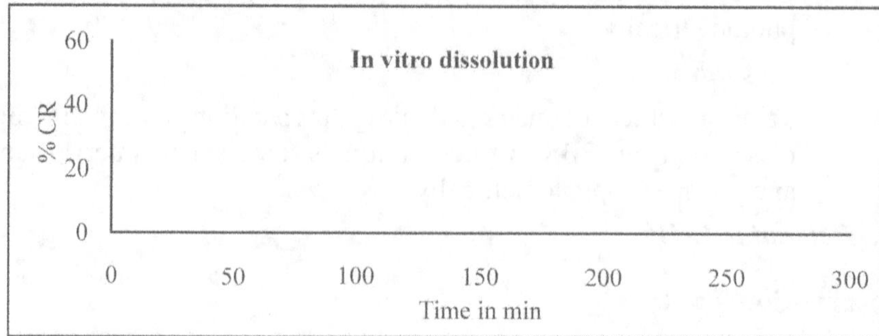

Rate of Absorption

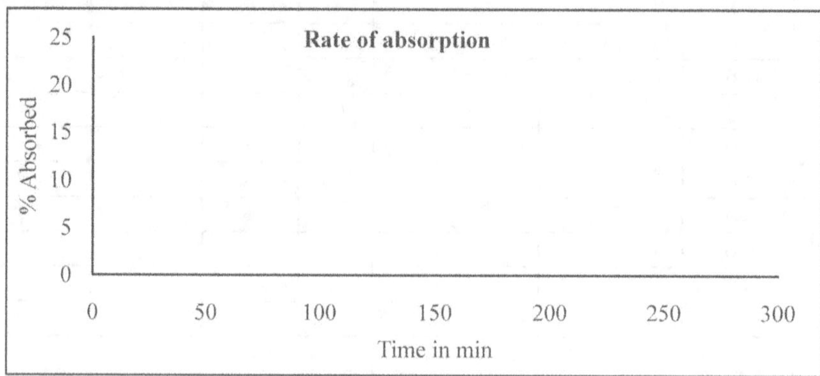

IVIVC

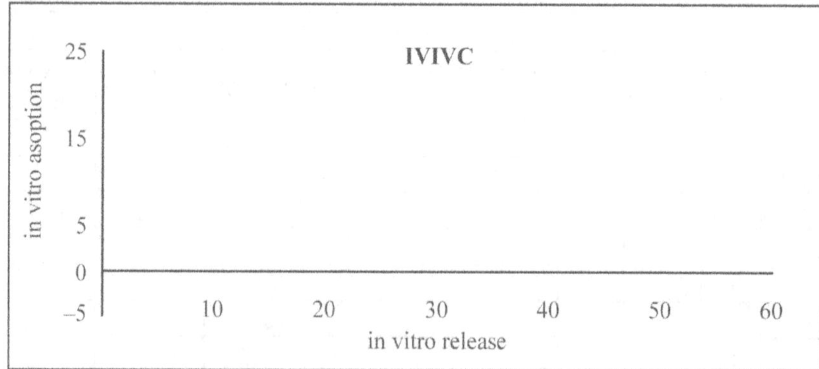

Experiment 33

Drug Release Kinetics

Drug dissolution is important test used to evaluate drug release of solid and semisolid dosage forms. This test is developed for quantification of the amount and extent of drug release from dosage forms. The values that are obtained from the dissolution study can be quantitatively analyzed by using different mathematical formulae. Because qualitative and quantitative changes in a formulation may alter release of drug and *in vivo* performance, developing tools that facilitate product development by reducing the necessity of bio-studies is always desirable. Thus, mathematical models can be developed.

This development requires the comprehension of all phenomena affecting drug release kinetics and this has a very important value in the formulation optimization. The model can be simply thought as a 'mathematical metaphor of some aspects of reality'. For this generality, mathematical modeling is widely employed in different disciplines such as genetics, medicine, psychology, biology, economy and obviously engineering and technology. Model dependent methods are based on different mathematical functions, which describe the dissolution profile. Once a suitable function has been selected, the dissolution profiles are evaluated depending on the derived model parameters. To compare dissolution profiles between two drug products model dependent (curve fitting), statistical analysis and model independent methods can be used.

The advancement in material design and engineering has led to the rapid development of novel materials with increasing complexity and functions. Both non-degradable and degradable polymers have found wide applications in the controlled delivery field. Studies on drug release kinetics provide important information into the function of material systems. To elucidate the detailed transport mechanism and the structure-function relationship of a material system, it is critical to bridge the gap between the macroscopic data and the transport behavior at the molecular level. Understanding the structure-function relationship of the material system is key to the successful design of a delivery system for a particular application. Moreover, developing complex polymeric matrices requires more robust mathematical models to elucidate the solute transport mechanisms. Many mathematical models have been used to design a number of simple and complex drug delivery systems and to predict the overall release behavior. They allow the measurement of some important physical parameters and resorting to model fitting on experimental release data. It is very important to know how to use these equations to understand the different factors that affect the release velocity and how the dissolution behaviors can vary and influence the efficiency or the therapeutic regimen of patients. The various mathematical models include zero order, first order, Higuchi, Hixson–Crowell, Ritger–Peppas–Kormeyers, Brazel–Peppas, Baker–Lonsdale, Hopfenberg, Weibull and Peppas–Sahlin.

Object

Determine drug release kinetics from tablet formulation.

References

1. Gao P, Nixon PR and Skoug JW. Diffusion in HPMC gels. II. Prediction of drug release rates from hydrophilic matrix extended-release dosage forms. Pharm. Res., 1995, 12: 965-971.

2. Shoaib MH, Tazeen J, Merchant A and Yousuf R. Evaluation of drug release kinetics from ibuprofen matrix tablets using HPMC, Pak. J. Pharm. Sci., 19(2), 2006, 119-124.

Requirements

Chemicals: Ibuprofen, HPMC K4M, Avicel PH-101, magnesium stearate etc.

Glassware etc.: Beaker, mortar pestle, glass rod, funnel, measuring cylinder, pipette etc.

Principle

Hydrophillic polymer matrix systems are widely used in oral controlled drug delivery systems because of their flexibility to obtain a desirable drug release profile, cost effectiveness, and broad regulatory acceptance. Drug release from hydrophillic matrices is known to be a complex interaction between dissolution, diffusion and erosion mechanisms. Hydroxypropyl methylcellulose (HPMC) is the first choice for formulation of hydrophilic matrix system, providing robust mechanism, choice of viscosity grades, nonionic nature, consistent reproducible release profiles, cost effectiveness and utilization of existing conventional equipment and methods. Water penetration, polymer swelling, drug dissolution, drug diffusion and matrix erosion from dosage form is controlled by the hydration of HPMC, which forms the gel barrier through which the drug diffuses.　HPMC is a hydrophillic polymer that swells to a significant extent upon contact with water.

The mathematical description of the entire drug release process is rather difficult, because of the number of physical characteristics that must be taken into consideration. These include the diffusion of water into the HPMC matrix, HPMC swelling, drug diffusion out of the device, polymer dissolution, axial and radial transport in a 3-dimensional system, concentration dependent diffusivities of the species, moving boundaries, and changing matrix dimensions, porosity and composition. Each model makes certain assumptions and due to these assumptions, the applicability of the respective models is restricted to certain drug–polymer systems.

Formula

S. No.	Name of Ingredient	Quantity Given (%w/w)	Quantity Taken (%w/w)
1	Ibuprofen	67	
2	HPMC	20	
3	Avicel	11	
4	Magnesium stearate	01	

Procedure

1. Transfer accurately weighed ingredients in geometric dilution method to a polythene bag and mix.
2. Compress by direct compression using a punching machine.
3. Evaluate the tablet on various parameters of weight, weight variation, thickness, hardness, friability, disintegration test.
4. For the dissolution test to determine rate kinetics, use USP apparatus Type II. Maintain at $37 \pm 0.5°C$ and 50 rpm rotation speed.
5. Use 900 ml of PBS pH 7.2 as the dissolution media for 12 hrs.
6. Collect aliquots at regular intervals, replace with fresh, prewarmed buffer, filter, dilute if required and analyse using UV spectrophotometer at 221nm.

Data Analysis

To analyse the *in vitro* release data various kinetic models can be used to describe the release kinetics. The zero-order rate Eq. (1) describes the systems where the drug release rate is independent of its concentration the first order Eq. (2) describes the release from system where release rate is concentration dependent. The release of drugs from insoluble matrix is a square root of time dependent process based on Fickian diffusion Eq. (3). The Hixson-Crowell cube root law Eq. (4) describes the release from systems where there is a change in surface area and diameter of particles or tablets.

$$C = k_o t \qquad \qquad .....(1)$$

Where, K_0 is zero-order rate constant expressed in units of concentration/time and t is the time.

$$LogC \ LogC \ kt / 2.303 \ o = - \qquad .....(2)$$

Where, C_0 is the initial concentration of drug and K is first order constant.

$$Q = K_t 1/ 2 \qquad \qquad .....(3)$$

Where, K is the constant reflecting the design variables of the system.

$$Q_0^{1/3} - Q_t^{1/3} = K_{HC} \ t \qquad \qquad .....(4)$$

Where, Qt is the amount of drug released in time t, Q0 is the initial amount of the drug in tablet and KHC is the rate constant for Hixson-Crowell rate equation.

Draw the following plots:

  (a) Cumulative % drug release vs. Time (zero order kinetic model)
  (b) Log cumulative of % drug remaining vs. Time (first order kinetic model)
  (c) Cumulative % drug release vs. Square root of time (Higuchi model)
  (d) Log cumulative % drug release vs. log time (Korsmeyer model)
  (e) Cube root of drug % remaining in matrix vs. time (Hixson-Crowell cube root law)

To determine the mechanism of drug release

Use Korsmeyer method of a simple relationship which describes drug release from a polymeric system Eq. (5). To find out the mechanism of drug release, first 60% drug release data is fitted in Korsmeyer–Peppas model:

$$Mt \ M = Kt \infty / \qquad \qquad .....(5)$$

Where Mt / M∞ is fraction of drug released at time t, k is the rate constant and n is the release exponent. The n value is used to characterize different release mechanisms for cylindrical shaped matrices.

  0.45 Fickian diffusion

  $0.45 < n < 0.89$ Anomalous (non-Fickian) diffusion

  0.89 Case-II transport

  $n > 0.89$ Super case-II transport

Observations

Physicochemical parameters of the tablets

Formulation	Parameters				
	Weight variation %	Thickness mm	Friability %	Hardness kg	Drug Content %
Formulation1					
Formulation2					

Release parameters and kinetic estimation

Zero Order		First Order		Higuchi		Korsemeyer Peppas			Hixon-Crowel	
r^2	$k_0(h^{-1})$	r^2	$k_1(h^{-1})$	r^2	$k_H(h^{-1/2})$	r^2	n	$k_{KP}(h^{-n})$	r^2	$k_{HC}(h^{-1/3})$

Preformulation Studies

Preformulation testing is the first step in the rational development of dosage forms. It can be defined as an investigation of physical and chemical property of a drug substance alone and when combined with excipients. It is also the phase of research and development in which preformulation studies characterize physical and chemical properties of a drug molecule in order to develop safe, effective and stable dosage form.

Preformulation evolved in the late 1950s and early 1960s as a result of a shift in emphasis in industrial pharmaceutical product development. It was improvement in analytical methods that spurred the first programs that might bear the name "preformulation". The overall objective of preformulation testing is to generate information useful to the formulator in developing stable and bioavailable dosage forms which can be mass-produced.

During the early development of a new drug substance, the synthetic chemist, alone or in co-operation with specialists in other disciplines including preformulation, may record some data which can be appropriately considered as preformulation data. Before starting the preformulation studies we should know the properties of the drug, potency relative to the competitive products and the dosage form, literature search providing stability and decay data, the proposed route of drug administration, literature search regarding the formulation approaches, bioavailability and pharmacokinetics of chemically related drugs. It also includes preliminary investigations and molecular optimization by the drug should be tested to determine the magnitude of each Suspected problem area (Step I), if a deficiency is detected, a molecular modification should be done (Step II). To overcome this deficiency molecular modification is done be salts, prodrugs, solvates, polymorphs or even new analogues. The dissolution rate of a salt form of a drug is generally quite different from that of the parent compound. Sodium and potassium salts of weak organic acids and hydrochloride salts of weak organic bases dissolve much more readily than do the, respective free acids or bases. After completion of preformulation evaluation of new drug candidates, a comprehensive report be prepared highlighting the pharmaceutical problems associated with molecules. It helps in developing phase I formulations and in preparing regulatory documents and aid in developing subsequent drug candidates. If, drug is found satisfactory sufficient quantity is synthesized to perform initial toxicity studies, initial analytical work and initial preformulation. Once past initial toxicity, phase I (clinical toxicology) begins for actual formulations. After that phase II and III clinical testing begins, and during this phase an order of magnitude formula is finalized. After completion of all above, an NDA is submitted and after approval of NDA, production can start.

Object

Establish preformulation parameters of given drug sample.

References

1. Gaud R.S., Gupta G.D., In; Practical Physical Pharmacy, CBS publisher and distributor, Ed-1, 2003, Pg No.: 112, 148.
2. Mohanta G.P., Manna P.K., Physical pharmacy, Practical text, Pharma book syndicate, Ed-1, 2006, Pg No. 27.

Theory

Preformulation studies are an essential component of drug development wherein it supports development of formulations, for different stages of clinical trials. The word preformulation is composed of two words pre and formulation. Activities done prior to formulation development are called as preformulation studies. It provides the scientific basis for formulation development.

Requirements

Chemicals: Paracetamol, salicylic acid, liquid paraffin, conc. HCl, NaOH, octanol, benzene, methanol, ethanol, phenolphthalein, ether, talc.

Glassware: Beaker, burette, conical flask, capillary tube, funnel, glass rod, measuring cylinder, pipette, separating funnel, test tube, thermometer, thiele's tube, volumetric flask, bulk density apparatus, tapped density apparatus, UV spectrophotometer.

Procedure

1. **Melting Point:**
   - Take Thiele's tube and clean it. Fill liquid paraffin in thiele's tube.
   - Heat seal capillary at one side and fill dry drug sample into it.

- Tie this capillary with thermometer. Dip capillary with thermometer in thiele's tube.
- Heat thiele's tube from elongated portion. Note point at which drug get melt down.

2. Solubility:

- Take 25 mL of distilled water in beaker and add benzoic acid to it up to saturated solution formed. Cool beaker at room temperature.
- Take 5 mL of supernatant and titrate against 0.1 N NaOH taking phenolphthalein as indicator. Repeat procedure 3 times. Note down the readings.

3. P_{ka}:

- Prepare 0.5% w/v solution of salicylic acid in methanol. Take 10 mL of salicylic acid solution in conical flask.
- Titrate it against 0.5 N NaOH solution using methyl red as indicator to complete neutralization. Note down the reading.
- Similarly take 10 mL of 0.5% w/v salicylic acid in methanol into a flask and titrate against 0.5 N NaOH solution to the half of the NaOH consumed previously.
- Note the pH of the solution.

4. Partition coefficient:

- Add excess amount of benzoic acid in 110 mL of benzene, Use this solution as stock solution.
- Prepare four sample A, B, C and D using 50:40:10 ratio of water: stock: benzene similarly prepare 50:30:20, 50:20:30 and 50:10:40 solutions.
- Take 10 mL of above solution and titrate against 0.1 N NaOH, note volume consumed.

1. Bulk Density

- Weigh 5gm of drug and fill in measuring cylinder, measure initial volume of talc.

2. Tapped Density

- Fit measuring cylinder in bulk density apparatus.
- Tap measuring cylinder about 100 times, measure final volume.

3. Angle of Repose

- Fix funnel in burette stand, Weigh accurately 2 gm of drug.
- Pass powder from measuring cylinder, measure height and diameter of pile.

4. Particle Size Distribution:

- Weigh accurately 2gm of powder and pour into sieve set.
- Do the sieving for 5 min, measure the weight of sample passed from each sieve.
- Plot the graph and do the calculations.

Formula

Bulk density = mass/initial volume

Tapped density = mass/final volume

Hausner's ratio = tapped density/bulk density

Angle of repose = $\tan^{-1}$H/R

Carr's index = tapped density – bulk density/tapped density × 100

Observation

1. Melting point
2. P_{ka}

Complete Neutralization

S. No.	Volume of drug solution	Volume of NaOH		pH
		Initial	Final	
1.	10 mL	0		
2.	10 mL	0		
3.	10 mL	0		
Half Neutralization				
1.	10 mL	0		

1. Solubility

S. No.	Temperature	Volume of NaOH		Total	Average
		Initial	Final		
1.	Room Temperature				
2.					
3.					

Partition coefficient

S. No.	Ratio	Layer	Burette reading		Total	Concentration
			Initial	Final		
1.						
2.						
3.						

$P = C_{oil}/C_{water}$

Angle of repose $= Tan^{-1}H/R$

S. No.	Height of Pile	Diameter	Average	Average Radius
1.				
2.				
3.				
4.				

Particle size distribution

S. No.	Sieve aperture	Average particle size (mm)	Wt of particle passed	% wt of particle passed	Cumulative % wt of particle passed	Cumulative undersized particle
1	10					
2	24					
3	80					

Experiment 35

Sterile Ophthalmic Preparations

Ophthalmic preparations are sterile liquid, semi-solid, or solid preparations intended for application to the conjunctiva, the conjunctival sac, or the eyelids. Sterility is a key issue in manufacture and use of ophthalmic products. Preservative selection is a critical activity in product design. Other important aspects requiring assessment in the manufacture of ophthalmic products include sterility, tonicity, pH, buffering, drug toxicity, solubility, stability, viscosity, aseptic filling, packaging and storage.

Microbial content or bioburden of the raw materials, in-process intermediates, and drug substance or active product ingredient are potential sources of contamination and require incoming testing of ingredients. Most ophthalmic products are sterilized by aseptic filtration through a 0.22-μm filter. Preservatives in the ophthalmic solution will, to varying degrees, bind or be adsorbed onto many common membrane filter materials. Most commercial liquid ophthalmic products are packaged in plastic containers fitted with nozzles for drop wise administration.

Plastic containers are generally sterilized by gamma irradiation or ethylene oxide. Facilities used to prepare ophthalmic preparations are required to operate within a controlled environment using HEPA filtration to minimize contact of airborne contamination with critical sites such as open product prior to application of closures, injection ports, and vial septa. Aseptic filling ophthalmic medications is typically achieved through the use of blow-fill-seal (BFS) technology in which product containers are formed from plastic granules on-line and then filled with drug solution and sealed in one operation. Blow-fill-seal-technology has a theoretically lower risk of microbial contamination compared with conventional aseptic filling. Quality control of these products includes traditional tests such as identification, potency, purity, impurities, sterility, and particulate matter and performance tests such as dissolution or drug release.

Physical or chemical instability will be demonstrated by noticeable changes in the dosage form such as changes in color, consistency, agglomerates, grittiness, emulsion breakdown, crystal growth, shrinking due to evaporation of water, or evidence of microbial growth. The finished product must also be subject to the sterility test and endotoxin tests.

The first contamination-related consideration is with the selection of the preservative and its efficacy. An ideal preservative is a rapidly effective and topically non-irritating. It may be a single antimicrobial agent or a mixture of such agents. Preservatives are designed to prevent the growth or to destroy microorganisms accidentally introduced into the product when the container is opened during use. Preservatives are a necessary additive.

Object

Formulate and evaluate sterile ophthalmic preparations.

References

1. Nanjwade B, Sonaje, Manvi FV, Preparation and Evaluation of Eye-drops for the treatment of Bacterial Conjunctivitis, IJPI's Journal of Pharmaceutics and Cosmetology, 1:2 (2011), 43-49.
2. Gilman M. R., in Hayes A. W. eds, 'Skin and eye testing in animals,' Principles and methods of toxicology, Ravan Press, NY 1986, pp. 209-212.

Requirements

Chemicals: Ciprofloxacin hydrochloride USP, Dexamethasone IP, hydroxypropyl-β-cyclodextrin, Methocel and Benzalkonium chloride IP, distilled water etc.

Glassware: Volumetric flask, glass rod, beaker, funnel etc.

Principle

Bacterial infections of the eye often cause severe inflammation. This inflammation can prove to the destructive to ocular tissues and may lead to partial or total impairment of vision. In order to prevent this treatment should be started not only with antibiotics but also with anti-inflammatory agents such as steroids. The use of steroids concomitantly with antibiotics greatly improves the clinical outcome of bacterial infections of the eye.

In the present practical two types of eye drops are prepared viz. a clear solution and a suspension. Preparation of solution involved a fairly simple process. Preparation of the suspension is done after sterilization of ingredient separately and mixing them aseptically. EDTA was used as a chelating agent and Methocel as a viscosity-increasing agent. Sodium chloride was used to adjust the tonicity.

Procedure

(i)   0.3% w/v ciprofloxacin and 0.1% w/v dexamethasone ophthalmic solution

    1. Prepare weak acetate buffer IP

    2. Prepare the aseptic chamber and proceed for the following

        (a) Take the buffer in a volumetric flask and dissolve Ciprofloxacin hydrochloride, benzalkonium chloride, EDTA and sodium chloride in a part of it.

        (b) To the other part of the buffer, add hydroxypropyl-β-cyclodextrin and heat the solution to 90°C with stirring.

        (c) Dissolve Dexamethasone in this solution and subsequently add HPMC to it.

        (d) Mix the two solutions and make up the volume up to the required level using the buffer solution.

        (e) Sterilize the solution was sterilized by membrane filtration.

(ii) 0.3% w/v ciprofloxacin and 0.1% w/v dexamethasone ophthalmic suspension

    1. Prepare weak acetate buffer IP and sterilize by autoclaving

    2. Prepare the aseptic chamber and proceed for the following

        (a) Take the buffer and in a part of it dissolve Ciprofloxacin hydrochloride, EDTA and sodium chloride in it. Let it be Mixture A.

        (b) Dissolve HPMC and benzalkonium chloride in buffer and sterilize by autoclaving.

        (c) Take pre-sterilized dexamethasone (sterilized by autoclaving at 140°C for 3 hours in vacuum) and mix with sterile HPMC mucilage under aseptic condition (Mixture B).

        (d) Mix both the mixtures A and B with constant stirring, under vacuum and make up the volume with sterile acetate buffer.

(iii) Keep both the eye-drops formulation in pre-sterilized amber coloured type I glass vial which are closed with pre-sterilized LDPE stoppers and sealed with aluminium crimps.

Evaluation

(i)   Physicochemical evaluation

   1. Evaluate the ophthalmic solution for:

      (a)   Visual appearance- by observing the solution against white and black background under fluorescent light.

      (b)   Clarity- by observing the solution against white and black background under fluorescent light.

      (c)   pH- using digital pH meter.

      (d)   drug content – by assay as per IP.

      (e)   Resuspendability- Invert the container at the rate of about 8-10 times in a minute. The number of inversions required to completely re-suspend the settled dexamethasone particles is noted.

(ii)   Microbiological evaluation

Carry out the test for sterility as per guidelines given in USP 23 by membrane filtration method.

The effectiveness of antimicrobial preservative can be carried out as per guidelines given in USP 23 using the test microbes as. E. coli, S. aureus, P. aeruginosa, C. albicans and A. niger.

(iii)   Biological evaluation

Biological evaluation include test for eye irritation and the test for efficacy of the formulations.

Experiment 36

pH Partition Hypothesis

pH partition is the tendency for acids to accumulate in basic fluid compartments, and bases to accumulate in acidic compartments. The reason for this phenomenon is that acids become negatively electric charged in basic fluids, since they donate a proton. On the other hand, bases become positively electric charged in acid fluids, since they receive a proton. Since electric charge decrease the membrane permeability of substances, once an acid enters a basic fluid and becomes electrically charged, then it cannot escape that compartment with ease and therefore accumulates, and vice versa with bases.

The pH-partition hypothesis was proposed by Brodie and his associates (in 1957) to explain the influence of GI pH and drug pKa on the extent of drug transfer or drug absorption. According to this theory for drug compounds of molecular weight greater than 100 and those which are primarily transported across the membrane by passive diffusion, the process of absorption is governed by three important factors like:

1. The dissociation constant i.e., pKa of the drug.
2. The lipid solubility of the unionised drug i.e., partition coefficient (Ko/w).
3. pH at the absorption site. As most of the pharmaceutical drugs are weak electrolytes, their absorption will be chiefly determined by the extent to which the drug exists in unionized form at the site of absorption.

The above hypothesis of the theory was based on the following assumptions:

1. GIT is a simple lipoidal barrier to the transport of drugs.
2. Larger the fraction of unionised drug, faster is its absorption.
3. Greater the lipophilicity (Ko/w) of the unionised drug, better is the absorption.

The amount of the drug present in unionised form is a function of pKa of the drug and pH of the fluid at the absorption site. The pKa value for either the acidic or the basic drug indicates the amount of undissociated drug present available for absorption at the absorption site. The lower the pKa value of the acidic drug, stronger is the acid i.e., greater is the proportion of ionised form at a particular pH. Similarly, higher the pKa value of a basic drug, the stronger is the base. Thus, the relative amount of ionised and unionised drug in a solution at a particular pH and the percent of drug ionised at this pH is given by Henderson-Hasselbach Equations. However, the conditions of GIT are not same all through. So unchanged, ionised acid or base are best absorbed from the small intestine as a result of large surface area and more contact time. Literature works on drug absorption infers that the acidic drugs are best absorbed from the acidic gastric fluids and basic drugs are best absorbed from the alkaline environment.

Object

Determine effect of different pH condition on solubility of a weekly acidic or basic drug and study pH partition hypothesis.

References

1. Tipnis HP, Nagarsenkar MS, Introduction to biopharmaceutics and pharmacokinetics, Nirali prakashan, 2003, 68-85.
2. Lieberman HA, Lachman L and Shwartz JB, pharmaceutical dosage forms, tablets, vol 2, 438-469.

Requirements

Chemicals: Salicylic acid n-octanol, Hydrochloric acid, Sodium hydroxide, Potassium chloride, potassium hydrogen phthalate, potassium dihydrogen phosphate, ferric chloride.

Glassware: Pipette, separating funnels, volumetric flasks, funnel etc.

Apparatus etc.: Digital electronic balance, UV/Visible spectrophotometer, etc.

Principle

Partitioning is the ability of a drug to distribute in two immiscible systems. The ability of drug to permeate across biological membranes has traditionally been evaluated using its partitioning in octanol [representing lipid membrane] and water system. Occasionally, other organic solvents like chloroform, ether and hexane have been used as lipid solvents instead of octanol to evaluate drug partitioning behaviour. When a drug is placed in an immiscible system comprising of octanol and water, the drug distributes in each solvent and eventually reaches equilibrium. The ratio of drug concentration in each phase is termed its distribution coefficient or partition coefficient.

The pKa of the drug determines the degree of ionization at a particular pH and only unionized drug with sufficient lipid solubility is absorbed into the systemic circulation. For optimum absorption, the drug should have sufficient aqueous solubility to dissolve in the GIT at the absorption site and lipid solubility should be high enough to facilitate drug partitioning of the drug into the lipoidal membrane and into systemic circulation. The partition coefficient [log p] value in the range of 1 to 3 has good passive absorption lipid membranes, and log p is greater or less than 3 have often poor transport characteristics. Highly non-polar molecules form a depot. The relationship between distribution coefficient and the apparent lipid-water partition (APC) can be estimated from the in vitro data of APC.

Formula $APC = (C_1 - C_2).a/ C_2b$

Where,

C1 = drug concentration in aqueous phase before equilibrium

C2 = drug concentration in aqueous phase after equilibrium

A = volume of aqueous phase

B = volume of organic phase

Procedure

Construction of calibration curve for salicylic Acid by visible spectroscopic method

Preparation of salicylic acid primary stock solution [1000μg/mL]

Weigh accurately 100mg of salicylic acid and transferred in to 100mL volumetric flask. Add small quantity of distilled water and shake the solution thoroughly to dissolve salicylic acid and make up the volume

Preparation of salicylic acid secondary stock solution [400 μg /mL]

Transfer 40 mL of the primary stock solution to 100mL volumetric flack and make up the volume with distilled water.

Preparation of working standard solution

Prepare a series of dilute solutions of 20,40,60,80, and 100μg/mL from the above secondary stock solution by taking 0.5, 1, 1.5, 2, 2.5mL & add 5mL of 4% ferric nitrate solution and finally the volume is make up to10mL with distilled water. Keep the solution aside for 10 minutes to develop a color. Measure the absorbance at 547nm in UV/Visible spectrometer. Plot a graph by taking concentration (μg /mL) on x- axis and absorbance on y- axis. This plot gives a straight line and the linearity can be determined using y = mx + c formula. Calculate the coefficient of determination, **R2** value, slope **m** and intercept **c.**

Determination of partition coefficient

(a) Prepare buffers with pH 4, 6.8 and 7.4.

(b) Take thoroughly cleaned and dried 6 numbers of separating funnels and label them S1, S2, S3.

(c) Take 25mL of n – octanol and 25mL of acid phthalate buffer pH 2.2in S1 separating funnel, 100mg of salicylic acid is added and shaken for one hour.

(d) From this mixture remove one mL of aqueous layer and transfer to 100mL volumetric flask. Finally make up to 100mL with distilled water.

(e) Take 5mL of the above solution then add 5mL of 4% ferric nitrate solution.

(f) Keep the solution aside for 10minutes to develop colour.

(g) Measure the absorbance at 547nm using 5mL of water with 5mL of 4% ferric nitrate solution as blank.

(h) To the separating funnel S2, S3 add the respective buffer with varying pH and repeat the same procedure.

(i) From the absorbance at different pH, calculate the concentration of salicylic acid at different pH.

Observations

Calibration curve for salicylic acid

S. No.	Drug concentration in µg/mL	Stock solution volume in mL	Volume of 4% Ferric chloride solution	Volume of distilled water	Absorbance
1	0	0	5	5.0	
2	20	0.5	5	4.5	
3	40	1.0	5	4.0	
4	60	1.5	5	3.5	
5	80	2.0	5	3.0	
6	100	2.5	5	2.5	

Partition coefficient determination

S. No.	Buffer pH	Absorbance	concentration µg/mL	Amount of drug in 25 mL of n-octanol (x)	Amount of drug in 25 mL of n-octanol (y)	Partition coefficient y/x
1	4.0					
2	6.8					
3	7.4					

Enteric Tablets

An enteric coating is a polymer barrier applied on oral medication that prevents its dissolution or disintegration in the gastric environment. This helps by either protecting drugs from the acidity of the stomach, the stomach from the detrimental effects of the drug, or to release the drug after the stomach (usually in the upper tract of the intestine). Some drugs are unstable at the acid gastric pH and need to be protected from degradation. Enteric coating is also an effective method to obtain drug targeting (such as gastro-resistant drugs). Enteric coating may also be used during studies as a research tool to determine drug absorption. Enteric coated medications pertain to the "delayed action" dosage form category. Tablets, mini-tablets, pellets and granules (usually filled into capsule shells) are the most common enteric-coated dosage forms.

Most enteric coatings work by presenting a surface that is stable at the highly acidic pH found in the stomach but breaks down rapidly at a higher pH. For example, they will not dissolve in the gastric acids of the stomach (pH ~3), but they will in the alkaline (pH 7–9) environment present in the small intestine. The time required for an enteric-coated dosage form to reach the intestine mostly depends on the presence and type of food in the stomach. It varies from 30 minutes up to 7 hours, with an average time of 6 hours. Although some studies indicated that larger sized dosage forms may require additional time for gastric emptying, others suggested that the size, shape, or volume of the tablet possess no significant effects instead. Enteric coated granules emptying rate is, however, less affected by the presence of food and present the more uniform release and reproducible transit time typical of the multi particulate dispersion. By preventing the drug from dissolving into the stomach, enteric coating may protect gastric mucosa from the irritating effects of the medication itself. When the drug reaches the neutral or alkaline environment of the intestine, its active ingredients can then dissolve and become available for absorption into the bloodstream. Drugs that have an irritant effect on the stomach, such as aspirin or potassium chloride, can be coated with a substance that will dissolve only in the small intestine. However, it has been shown that enteric coated aspirin may lead to incomplete inhibition of platelets. Materials used for enteric coatings include fatty acids, waxes, shellac, plastics, and plant fibers. The first form of gastro-resistant coating was introduced by Unna in 1884 in the form of keratin-coated pills, although it was later discovered that they weren't able to withstand gastric digestion. Salol was also used by Ceppi as one of the first forms of enteric coating. However, the first material that was extensively used as enteric coating agent was shellac, since its introduction in 1930.

Object

To perform enteric coating of tablets.

References

1. Lachman Leon, Liberman AH, Joseph HL Kanic, "The theory and practice of industrial pharmacy", 3rd edition published by Varghese 1987, 293-344.

2. Niazi SK: "Hand book of Pharmaceutical Manufacturing formulations, compressed solid Products, Volume 1, CRC Press, Florida, 284-287.

3. Lieberman, AH, Lachmann L, Joseph B, Schwartz, "Pharmaceutical dosage form", Volume 1 , 2nd edition , rev.& expanded: Tablet, 75-128.

Requirements

1. *Chemicals required:* Triethyl citrate (Eudraflex), Eudragit (Eudragit L 30D-55,) Dimethyl polysiloxane emulsion (30%), Polysorbate 80 NF, Iron oxide (red), Titanium dioxide (special coating grade), Talc powder, Purified water.

2. *Glassware required:* Pestle-Mortar, Beaker, Measuring Cylinder, Glass rod, Coating Pan, Sprayer and Sieves.

Formula

For Enteric Coating Solution

S. No.	Ingredient	Quantity (g/kg)
1	Purified water (distilled)	466.66
2	Talc powder	15.19
3	Titanium dioxide (special coating grade)	7.98
4	Iron oxide (red),	15.50
5	Polysorbate 80 NF	4.26
6	Dimethyl polysiloxane emulsion (30%),	0.15
7	Eudragit (Eudragit L 30D-55,)	476.00
8	Triethyl citrate (Eudraflex),	14.25

Theory

Tablet coating: Coating facilitates entire cover-up of the tablet surface with suitable coating materials like sugar, cellulose etc. The decision to coat a tablet is usually based on one or more of the following objectives:

1. To mask the taste, odour or colour of the drug.
2. To provide physical and chemical protection for the drug.
3. To control they release of the drug from the tablet.
4. To protect the drug from the gastric environment of the stomach with an acid resistant, enteric coating.
5. To incorporate another drug or formula adjuvant in the coating to avoid chemical incompatibilities or to provide sequential drug release.
6. To improve the pharmaceutical elegance by use of special colours and contrasting printing.

Enteric Coating

Enteric coating is a type of coating which does not permit the release of drug in acid medium of the medium of the stomach but in release the drug in Alkaline medium of the intestine.

Purpose of Enteric Coating:

(i) To prevent the decomposition of the drug in acid medium of the stomach.
(ii) To prevent the irritation of the drug in the stomach.
(iii) To obtain the required action in the intestine.

Material Used:

(i) Cellulose Acetate Phthalate (CAP).
(ii) Acrylates Polymers e.g. Eudragit L and Eudragit S.
(iii) Hydroxypropyl Methyl Cellulose Phthalate.
(iv) Polyvinyl Acetate Phthalate etc.

Procedure

Weigh the quantity of water needed. Take approximately 21.5% of the total quantity of water in a suitable mixing container. Add the talc powder and stir vigorously until well suspended (approximately 20 minutes). Add the following to the proceeding suspension, and mix thoroughly: titanium dioxide, iron oxide red, Tween 80 and dimethyl polysiloxane emulsion (30%).

Note: The pigments may require homogenizing with colloid, corrudum disc mill, or ball mill. Take the Eudragit L 30D-55 in a suitable mixing vessel and add the following with continuous mixing: homogenized pigment mixture from Step 2, Eudraflex (Trimethyl citrate) and the remaining quantity of water.

Note: When PEG 8000 is used as a plasticizer, it should be incorporated as a 10 % aqueous solution.

Coating Procedure

1. Tablet core loading –5 kg
2. Core size-9 mm biconvex
3. Quantity of suspension applied-1890 g
4. Quantity of solid/cm^2- 9 mg
5. Quantity of film-forming agent/cm^2-6 mg
6. Speed of coating pan-12 r/min
7. Spray nozzle-0.8 mm
8. Spraying pressure-2.0 bar
9. Type of spraying-continuous
10. Inlet air temperature-50°C
11. Outlet air temperature- approximately 30°C
12. Spraying time—approximately 60 min.
13. Spraying Rate- approximately 30 g/min

Result:

Experiment 38

Calibration and Validation of Laboratory Equipment

In every manufacturing facility, calibration and validation must be carried out to assure high quality of the product. These are done on a regular basis, rather them being just a one-off activity, and is required to meet all the regulatory requirements. Calibration can be defined as a process where a comparison is made between two entities: one whose value has to be measured and the other entity, known as the standard, which is used as the reference in the comparison. This process includes the adjustment of any instrument to bring it into alignment with the standard. Instrument Calibration is done regularly to make sure that they produce accurate results. It is important to calibrate:

- New instruments
- Before a critical measurement
- Instruments after a repair
- After the instrument has been used for a specific number of hours
- When there is a sudden change in the operating conditions or
- instrument environment
- When the measurements seem questionable

Validation is a process that ensures that a system, product or service consistently provides results within the acceptable criteria. The performance, quality, and other operating parameters are tested to verify that they comply with the necessary requirements. Usually, process validation is done by a third party to make sure that the buyer is given a product that meets the specifications, requirements, and accepted standards. Documented results must be produced at the end of the process. Equipment validation is a term used to describe a set of independent procedures that are used to check if a product meets the specifications and requirements of its intended purposes. Regulatory agencies around the world have strict requirements for quality, procedures, performance testing, safety checks and the like, for a wide range of products. Validation may be prospective, retrospective, concurrent or locational.

Calibration and validation are different in many aspects as

- Calibration is a process that ensures that accuracy is maintained in the measurements produced by your equipment while validation is a documented process that provides assurance that a product, service or system consistently provides results within the acceptable criteria.

- Calibration performance of any equipment is compared against a reference standard while there are no reference standards used in validation.

- Calibration assures accuracy of measurements while validation provides proof of consistency across all the processes, batches of products or methods being used.

- Instruments are periodically calibrated to identify if there is a 'drift' in the measurements and eliminate it through calibration while there are no such requirements for validation. It should be performed when you make any change in the existing system or when the revalidation period has reached.

Object

Calibration and validation of laboratory equipment.

1. Electronic Balance.

Operate the instrument as per respective Standard Operating Procedure.

1. Switch 'ON' the balance.
2. The display will blink with 8.8.8.8.8.8.
3. After few seconds, the display will show 0.00 g.
4. If display is not stable, press the TARE key & wait till the display shows 0.00 g.
5. Perform internal calibration and in Annexure-II

For Accuracy

1. Place 5 gm. on the weighing pan.
2. Note the weight.
3. Calculate the difference between the weight in certificate and observed weight.
4. Repeat the above steps using 50gm & 100 gm. weights.
5. Record the reading in Annexure-II.

For precision

1. Place 5 gm. in the weighing pan.

2. Note the weight.
3. Repeat the above two steps nine times.
4. Record the weight in Anenxure-I.
5. Calculate the Standard deviation.
6. Calculate the measurement uncertainty using following equation.

$$\text{Measurement uncertainty} = \frac{3 \times \text{SD}}{\text{Actual weight from certificate}}$$

Accuracy

Date	Internal Calibration	Observed weight	Difference

Limit

S. No.	Theoretical weight	Actual weights from certificates	Tolerance
1	5 gm. +/- 5mg		
2	50.0 gm. +/- 5mg		
3	100.0gm. +/- 5mg		

1. Hot air Oven

1. For the calibration of hot air oven use a standard thermometer ranging up to 300° C.
2. Start the calibration procedure after 1 hour of staring the oven.
3. Set the oven at desired temperature.
4. Put the standard thermometer for 30 minutes in upper shelf of oven and close the door of oven.
5. After 30 minutes open the door of oven and read the temperature of standard thermometer randomly and match the observed temperature of thermometer.
6. Repeat the above procedure by putting the thermometer in lower shelf for 30 minutes.
7. Record the observed temperature in calibration record of hot air oven as per annexure no. I

8. The observed temperature of thermometer in both shelves should be ± 2.0° C tolerance limit to the set temperature value.
9. Frequency: Once in a month.

2. Magnetic Stirrer

1. Place magnetic stirrer on a stable well-levelled surface.
2. Place stir bar at bottom of glass container.
3. Fill glass container with liquid.
4. Speed control knob completely turned anticlockwise.
5. Place glass container on centre of magnetic stirrer.
6. Turn magnetic stirrer On.
7. Achieved 3000 rpm stirring speed.
8. Turn magnetic stirrer Off.

3. Calibration of Centrifuge Apparatus

Procedure

Ensure that all connections of the instrument are proper. Operate the instrument as per the operating instructions. Use duly calibrated tachometer, digital thermometer and stop watch during calibration of the equipment.

Calibration of time

Set the time for five minutes using set parameters. Record the results by using digital stop watch. Repeat the test for ten minutes. Calibration of revolutions per minutes (RPM).

Fixed angle rotor

Set the RPM of rotor to 12000. Record the results by using tachometers. Set RPM of rotor to 6000. Record the results by using tachometers.

Swing out rotor

Set the RPM of rotor to 4000. Record the results by using tachometers. Set RPM of rotor to 2000. Record the results by using tachometers.

Calibration of temperature

Fixed angle rotor

Fill the two sample tubes with ethylene glycol and place it in sample holder. Set the parameters like temperature 5°C, RPM: 12000 and time 45 minutes.

Record the temperature of the sample solution by using digital thermometer.

Fill the two sample tubes with ethylene glycol and place it in sample holder. Set the parameters like temperature 10°C, RPM: 12000 and time

45 minutes. Record the temperature of the sample solution by using digital thermometer.

Fill the two sample tubes with ethylene glycol and place it in sample holder. Set the parameters like temperature 20°C, RPM: 12000 and time 45 minutes. Record the temperature of the sample solution by using digital thermometer.

Swing out rotor

Fill the two sample tubes with ethylene glycol and place it in sample holder. Set the parameters like temperature 5°C, RPM: 4000 and time 45 minutes.

Record the temperature of the sample solution by using digital thermometer.

Fill the two sample tubes with ethylene glycol and place it in sample holder. Set the parameters like temperature 10°C, RPM: 4000 and time 45 minutes. Record the temperature of the sample solution by using digital thermometer.

Fill the two sample tubes with ethylene glycol and place it in sample holder. Set the parameters like temperature 20°C, RPM: 4000 and time 45 minutes. Record the temperature of the sample solution by using digital thermometer.

Frequency

Perform the calibration after every six months. Record the results in the calibration record format.

4. Microscope

Place the stage micrometer (least count 0.01mm) on the slide holder (stage).

Replace the eye peace of microscope with the oculometer.

Fix the first mark of oculometer with first mark of stage micrometer using different magnifying lens (10x, 40x and 100x).

Calculate the least count of oculometer using formula given below for each (x) of objective.

Least count of Oculometer (μm) =

$$\frac{\text{No. of marks of stage micrometer} \times 0.01 \times 1000}{\text{No. of marks of oculometer matched with stage micrometer}}$$

5. pH Meter

1. Before starting the calibration make sure that the correct measurement mode is selected.

2. Wash the electrode thoroughly with de-Ionized water or a rinse solution. Do not wipe the electrode; this causes a build-up of electrostatic charge on the glass surface.

3. Maintain the temperature of the buffers to 25°C ± 2°C, unless otherwise specified in the individual monograph and dip the electrode along with the temperature sensor into the buffers.

4. Perform the five point calibration using standard buffers of pH 1.68, 5.01/5.00, 7.00/7.01, 10.00/10.01 and 12.45.

5. Dip the electrode into the calibration buffer. The end of the electrode must be completely immersed into the sample. Stir the electrode gently to create a homogeneous sample.

6. Press CAL/MEAS key to enter pH calibration mode.The CAL indicator will be shown. The primary display will show the measured reading while the smaller secondary display will indicate the pH standard buffer solution reading.

7. Wait for the measured pH value to stabilize.

8. Press HOLD/ENTER key to confirm calibration. The meter is now calibrated to the current buffer.

9. Fist rinse the electrode with de-ionized water, which is followed by next buffer solution and place it in the buffer solution.

10. Follow steps 5.5.5 to 5.5.9 for additional calibration points.

11. When all the calibration points set in the unit configuration set up are completed the meter returns to the measurement mode automatically. However, calibration can be terminated without completing the number of points as set in the unit configuration. It can be done by pressing CAL\MEAS to return to pH measurement mode. Record the calibration details and Temperature.

12. Change the calibration buffer every week or whenever required and record.

6. Thermometer

Each thermometer shall be numbered and identified by its number whenever it is used, either for calibration or for routine temperature measurements.

These thermometers are calibrated using following reference standards for their accuracy and record:

S. No.	Substances	Standard Thermometer Reading	Standard Melting Range
1	Vanillin		81 – 83°C
2	Acetanilide		114 – 116°C
3	Sulphanilamide		164.5 – 166.5°C
4	Caffeine		234 – 237°C

Any thermometer that breaks or does not respond to given temperature range should be discarded

7. UV-Vis Spectrophotometer

Calibration of UV-VIS Spectrophotometer is done in four steps.

(a) Control of Wave length

(b) Control of Absorbance

(c) Limit of Stray Light

(d) Resolution Power

1. Operate the instruments as per SOP.

2. Control of Wave length

Weight accurately 1.0 gm of Holmium Oxide and dissolve it in 1.4 M Perchloric acid solution. Make up to 25 mL with the same solvent.

Select the method file of CONTROL OF WAVE LENGTH in the instrument.

After selecting the file press Reference button for baseline correction.

Then fill the Cuvette with 1.4M Perchloric acid and put in the sample cubicle and press reference to zero.

After auto zero put the Holmium perchlorate solution in sample cubicle then press start key.

Scan it and verify the wavelength using absorption maxima of Holmium Perchlorate solution. The permitted tolerance is given in below table.

S. No.	Maxima Wave length (nm)	Tolerance (nm)
1.	241.15nm	240.15 nm to 242.15 nm
2.	287.15nm	286.15 nm to 288.15 nm
3.	361.5nm	360.50 nm to 362.50 nm
4.	536.3nm	533.30 nm to 539.30 nm

3. Control of Absorbance:

1. Dry a quantity of the Potassium dichromate by heating to constant weight at 130°C.

2. Weight accurately about 60 mg of dried potassium dichromate and dissolve it in 0.005M sulphuric acid solution. Make upto 1000 ml with the same solvent. Mark the solution as (A).

3. Weight accurately about 60 mg of dried potassium dichromate and dissolve it in 0.005M sulphuric acid solution. Make up to 100 ml with the same solvent. Mark the solution as (B).

4. Select the method file of CONTROL OF ABSORBANCE in the instrument.

5. After selecting the file press Reference button for baseline correction.

6. Then fill the Cuvette with 0.005M Sulphuric acid for blank and put in both sample cubicle and press reference to zero.

7. After auto zero put the Potassium Dichromate solution labeled as solution 'A' in sample cubicle then press start key taking absorbance individually for first four wavelengths mentioned in 'Table I'.

8. Now take absorbance at 430 nm for solution 'B'.

9. Note the absorption maxima of Potassium Dichromate solution at different wave length and calculate the absorbance, tolerance is given in below table.

Table 1

S. No.	Wavelength (nm)	Absorbance E (1%1cm)	Maximum tolerance
1.	235	124.5	122.9 to 126.2
2.	257	144.0	142.8 to 145.7
3.	313	48.6	47.0 to 50.3
4.	350	106.6	104.9 to 108.2
5.	430	15.9	15.7 to 16.1

4. Limit of Stray light

1. Dry a quantity of the Potassium chloride by heating to constant weight at 130°C.

2. Weight accurately 1.20 g of dried potassium chloride and dissolve it in 50 ml distilled water. Make up to 100 mL with the same solvent.

3. Select the method file of LIMIT OF STRAY LIGHT in the instrument.

4. After selecting the file press Reference button for baseline correction.

5. Check the absorbance of above solution using water as a blank at 200 nm.

6. Absorbance should be greater than 2.0

5. Resolution power

    1. Prepare 0.02%v/v solution of Toluene in Hexane UV.

    2. Select the method file of RESOLUTION POWER in the instrument.

    3. After selecting the file press Reference button for baseline correction.

    4. Measure the absorbance of above solution at 266 nm and 269 nm using Hexane UV as blank solution.

    5. The ratio of absorbance maxima at 269 nm to that of 266 nm minima should be more than 1.5

    6. Note down the report in the internal calibration certificate and in Instrument Logbook.

Experiment 39

Spectroscopic Estimation of Drugs

Object

Perform Spectrophotometric estimation of some commonly used drugs.

Principle

It is the branch of science dealing with the study of interaction between Electromagnetic radiation and matter. It is a most powerful tool available for the study of atomic and molecular structure/s and is used in the analysis of wide range of samples. Optical spectroscopy includes the region on electromagnetic spectrum between 100 Å and 400 μm is one of the most frequently employed technique in pharmaceutical analysis. It involves measuring the amount of ultraviolet or visible radiation absorbed by a substance in solution. Instrument which measure the ratio, or function of ratio, of the intensity of two beams of light in the U.V-Visible region are called Ultraviolet-Visible spectrophotometers. In qualitative analysis, organic compounds can be identified by use of spectrophotometer, if any recorded data is available, and quantitative spectrophotometric analysis is used to ascertain the quantity of molecular species absorbing the radiation. Spectrophotometric technique is simple, rapid, moderately specific and applicable to small quantities of compounds. The fundamental law that governs the quantitative spectrophotometric analysis is the Beer -Lambert law.

Beer's law: It states that the intensity of a beam of parallel monochromatic radiation decreases exponentially with the number of absorbing molecules. In other words, absorbance is proportional to the concentration.

Lambert's law: It states that the intensity of a beam of parallel monochromatic radiation decreases exponentially as it passes through a medium of homogeneous thickness. A combination of these two laws yields the Beer-Lambert law.

Beer-lambert law: When beam of light is passed through a transparent cell containing a solution of an absorbing substance, reduction of the intensity of light may occur. Mathematically, Beer- Lambert law is expressed as

$$A = a\ b\ c$$

Where,   A = absorbance or optical density

a = absorptivity or extinction coefficient

b = path length of radiation through sample (cm)

c = concentration of solute in solution.

Both b and a are constant so a is directly proportional to the concentration c.

When c is in gm/100 mL, then the constant is called A (1%, 1 cm).

Quantification of medicinal substance using spectrophotometer may carried out by preparing solution in transparent solvent and measuring its absorbance at suitable wavelength. The wavelength normally selected is wavelength of maximum absorption (λ_{max}), where small error in setting the wavelength scale has little effect on measured absorbance. Ideally, concentration should be adjusted to give an absorbance of approximately 0.9, around which the accuracy and precision of the measurements are optimal.

The assay of single component sample, which contains other absorbing substances, is then calculated from the measured absorbance by using one of three principal procedures. They are, use of standard absorptivity value, calibration graph and single or double point standardization. In standard absorptive value method, the use of standard A (1%, 1 cm) or E values are used in order to determine its absorptivity. It is advantageous in situations where it is difficult or expensive to obtain a sample of the reference substance. In calibration graph method, the absorbances of a number of standard solutions of the reference substance at concentrations encompassing the sample concentrations are measured and a calibration graph is constructed. The concentration of the analyte in the sample solution is read from the graph as the concentration corresponding to the absorbance of the solution. The single point standardization procedure involves the measurement of the absorbance of a sample solution and of a standard solution of the reference substance. The concentration of the substances in the sample is calculated from the proportional relationship that exists between absorbance and concentration.

$$C_{test} = (A_{test} \times C_{std})/A_{std}$$

Where, C_{test} and C_{std} are the concentrations in the sample and standard solutions respectively and A_{test} and A_{std} are the absorbances of the sample and standard solutions respectively. For assay of substance/s in multi component samples by spectrophotometer; the following methods are being used routinely, which includes

- Simultaneous equation method
- Derivative spectrophotometric method
- Absorbance ratio method (Q-Absorbance method)
- Difference spectrophotometry
- Solvent extraction method

1. UV Spectrophotometric estimation of Paracetamol

Paracetamol standard drug, marketed paracetamol tablets, analytical grade methanol and water Solvent- Methanol and water (15:85, v/v).

Standard preparation: Dissolve 100 mg drug in 150 mL methanol and shake well. Add 850 mL of water to adjust the volume up to 1000 mL (100 ppm). From that take 5 mL and adjust volume.

Test preparation: Take 20 tablets, weigh and powder. Weigh powdered tablet equivalent to 100 mg of Paracetamol in a 100 mL volumetric flask, add 15 mL of methanol and shake well to dissolve. Now add 85 mL of water to adjust the volume to 100mL. Withdraw 1 mL of solution in 100 mL volumetric flask and adjust volume to 100 mL.

Instrumentation: UV-Visible double beam spectrophotometer with matched quartz cells (1 cm).

Selection of wavelength: Scan standard solution in UV spectrophotometer between 200 nm to 400 nm on spectrum mode, using diluents as a blank. The λ max of Paracetamol is 247 nm.

UV Spectrophotometric estimation of Metoclopramide hydrochloride.

Metoclopramide hydrochloride standard drug, analytical grade methanol and water.

Solvent- Methanol

Standard preparation: Dissolve 100 mg drug in 100 mL methanol and shake well. Dilute suitably to get dilutions of standard in the concentration range 0-30 µg/mL.

Instrumentation: UV-Visible double beam spectrophotometer with matched quartz cells (10 mm).

Selection of wavelength: Scan standard solution in UV spectrophotometer between 200 nm to 400 nm on spectrum mode, using diluents as a blank. The λ max of Metoclopramide hydrochloride is 275 nm.

UV Spectrophotometric estimation of Zaltoprofen.

Zaltoprofen standard drug, analytical grade methanol and distilled water.

Solvent- Methanol and water

Standard preparation: Accurately 10 mg of drug and transfer to 100mL volumetric flask. Add 20 mL of methanol and dissolve by sonication for 10 min. Make up the volume with distilled water. Then, dilute suitably to get working standard of concentration 10µg/mL.

Instrumentation: Instrumentation- UV-Visible double beam spectrophotometer with matched quartz cells (10 mm).

Selection of wavelength: Scan standard solution in UV spectrophotometer between 200 nm to 400 nm on spectrum mode, using diluents as a blank. The λ max of Zaltoprofen is 227 nm.

UV Spectrophotometric estimation of Ciprofloxacin hydrochloride.

Ciprofloxacin hydrochloride, distilled water.

Solvent- Distilled water

Standard preparation: Weigh accurately 100 mg of the drug and dissolve it in 10 mL of distilled water in a volumetric flask. Shake well and make up the volume with distilled water. Dilute suitably to get concentration range of 2, 4, 6, 8, and 10µg/mL with distilled water.

Instrumentation: Instrumentation- UV-Visible double beam spectrophotometer with matched quartz cells (10 mm).

Selection of wavelength: Scan standard solution in UV spectrophotometer between 200 nm to 400 nm on spectrum mode, using diluents as a blank. The λ max of Ciprofloxacin hydrochloride is 274 nm.

UV Spectrophotometric estimation of Diclofenac sodium.

Diclofenac sodium, distilled water.

Solvent- Distilled water

Standard preparation: Weigh accurately 100 mg of the drug and dissolve it in 10 mL of distilled water in a volumetric flask. Shake well and make up the volume with distilled water. Dilute suitably to get concentration range of 5, 10, 15, 20, and 25µg/mL with distilled water.

Instrumentation: Instrumentation- UV-Visible double beam spectrophotometer with matched quartz cells (10 mm).

Selection of wavelength: Scan standard solution in UV spectrophotometer between 200 nm to 400 nm on spectrum mode, using diluents as a blank. The λ max of Diclofenac sodium is 276 nm.

Thin Layer Chromatography Estimation of Drugs

Object

Perform Thin layer chromatographic estimation of some commonly used drugs.

Principle

Thin-layer chromatography (TLC) is a chromatography technique used to separate non-volatile mixtures. Thin-layer chromatography is performed on a sheet of glass, plastic, or aluminium foil, which is coated with a thin layer of adsorbent material, usually silica gel, aluminium oxide (alumina), or cellulose. This layer of adsorbent is known as the stationary phase. After the sample has been applied on the plate, a solvent or solvent mixture (known as the mobile phase) is drawn up the plate via capillary action. Because different analytes ascend the TLC plate at different rates, separation is achieved. The mobile phase has different properties from the stationary phase. For example, with silica gel, a very polar substance, non-polar mobile phases such as heptane are used. The mobile phase may be a mixture, allowing chemists to fine-tune the bulk properties of the mobile phase. After the experiment, the spots are visualized. Often this can be done simply by projecting ultraviolet light onto the sheet; the sheets are treated with a phosphor, and dark spots appear on the sheet where compounds absorb the light impinging on a certain area. Chemical processes can also be used to visualize spots; anisaldehyde, for example, forms coloured adducts with many compounds, and sulfuric acid will char most organic compounds, leaving a dark spot on the sheet.

To quantify the results, the distance travelled by the substance being considered is divided by the total distance travelled by the mobile phase. (The mobile phase must not be allowed to reach the end of the stationary phase.) This ratio is called the retardation factor (R_f). In general, a substance whose structure resembles the stationary phase will have low R_f, while one that has a similar structure to the mobile phase will have high retardation factor. Retardation factors are characteristic but will change depending on the exact condition of the mobile and stationary phase. TLC plates are usually commercially available, with standard particle size ranges to improve reproducibility. They are prepared by mixing the adsorbent, such as silica gel, with a small amount of inert binder like calcium sulphate (gypsum) and water. This mixture is spread as a thick slurry on an unreactive carrier sheet, usually glass, thick aluminium foil, or plastic. The resultant plate is dried and activated by heating in an oven for thirty minutes at 110 °C. The thickness of the absorbent layer is typically around 0.1 – 0.25 mm for analytical purposes and around 0.5 – 2.0 mm for preparative TLC.

Thin Layer Chromatography of Amino Acids

Leucine, alanine, methionine, valine, serine, n butanol, acetic acid, distilled water, ninhydrin's reagent.

Solvent system- Mix n-butanol, acetic acid (purity 98 – 100 %) and distilled water in volume ratio 5:1:5. Stir for 10 minutes, then let the layers separate. Use upper layer as eluent.

Dissolve 0.3 g of ninhydrin in 100 mL n-butanol. Add 3 mL of glacial acetic acid.

Standard preparation- 0.02 M solutions of amino acids (leucine, methionine, alanine and serine). Dissolve 0.026 g leucine, 0.030 g methionine, 0.018 g alanine and 0.021 g serine in distilled water and bring the volume to 10mL.

Instrumentation- Chromatography chamber with lid.

Dip the capillary into solution and touch the prepared location on chromatographic paper. The spot on the paper should not be bigger than 2-3 mm. After application of samples let the spots dry.

Insert the chromatographic paper into the pre-saturated chromatography chamber and cover with the lid. Check if the paper reaches the eluent surface. Elution is stopped when the solvent front has travelled up the plate until 7-10 mm from the lid. Remove the paper from elution chamber and place it on a sheet of filter paper. After 2-3 minutes mark the eluent front with pencil and dry the paper in oven. When the paper is dry, take it into the fume hood and spray it with solution of ninhydrin until the paper is slightly damp. Chromatographic paper and the paper supporting it should lie at 45° angle while spraying. The chromatographic paper is again put in the drying oven for 15 min to speed up the reactions. Use the time to wash the gloves (let the gloves be on until washed). Use distilled water to rinse the capillaries and put into oven for drying. Pour the eluent from the elution chamber into residues bottle and let the chamber dry. Remove chromatographic paper from drying in the oven, draw the contours and centers of the chromatographic bands. Calculate RF values by the method described above. Compare retention of standard substances and components in sample and determine which amino acids were present in the sample.

Thin Layer Chromatography of Paracetamol

Paracetamol, Ethanol (99.8%), acetone, chloroform, ammonia and distilled water.

Solvent system- chloroform + acetone + ammonia (25%) in ration of 8:2:0.1.

Standard preparation- Dissolve paracetamol in ethanol to get the standard solution.

Instrumentation- Densitometer with TLC Scanner, Spectrophotometer, TLC plates: 10×20 cm glass plates precoated with 0.20 mm layers of silica gel, 5 µL micropipettes, chromatographic chambers.

Prewash the plates with methanol and dry overnight at room temperature. Activate at 120°C for 10 min in a hot air oven. Apply the samples and keep in the chamber for run. Allow sufficient running of the solvent front, allow the plates to dry and study.

Densitometric and spectrodensitometric investigations can be done using a TLC Scanner operated in the absorbance mode. The radiation source in it is a deuterium lamp emitting a continuous UV spectrum between 190 and 450 nm. Perform densitometric scanning at multiwavelength in the range of 200 to 400 nm, at wavelength intervals of 50 nm at each step. Finally, densitometric scanning, for quantitative determination of acetaminophen, is done at absorption maximum of acetaminophen equal to 248 nm.

FTIR of Common Drugs

1. Paracetamol

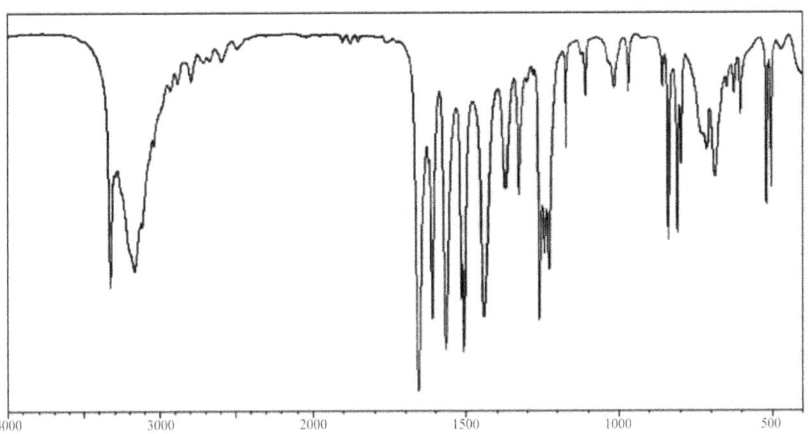

3326	30	1667	4	1373	63	1108	77	716	62
3165	33	1624	60	1329	52	970	77	689	57
3149	37	1611	21	1261	21	858	21	650	79
3114	44	1667	14	1244	37	839	41	626	77
3036	64	1516	26	1238	46	809	46	605	72
2930	77	1509	19	1226	34	787	60	521	49
2796	79	1444	22	1173	64	729	66	604	63

2. Omeprazole

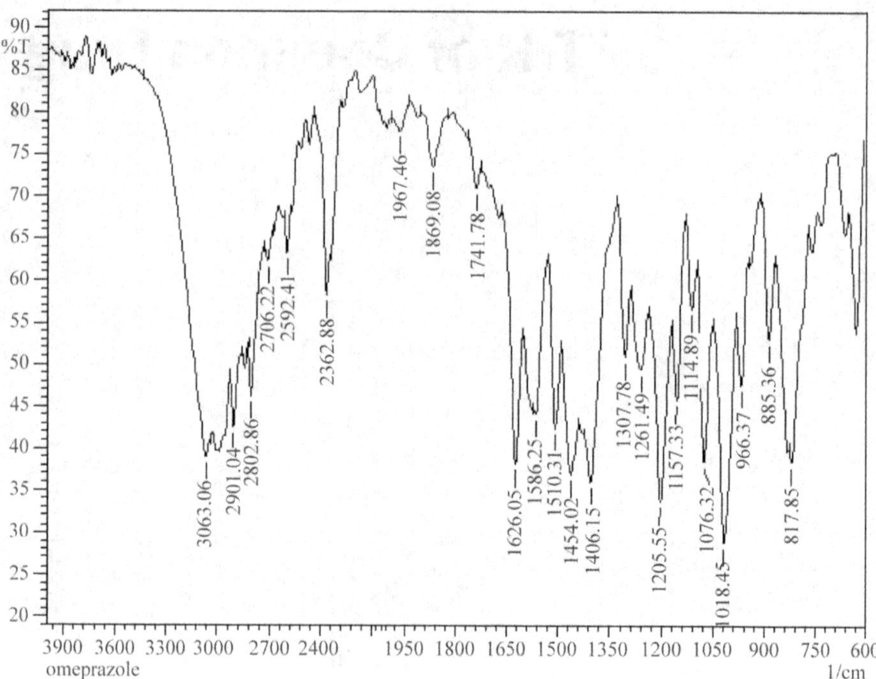

3. Clindamycin hydrochloride

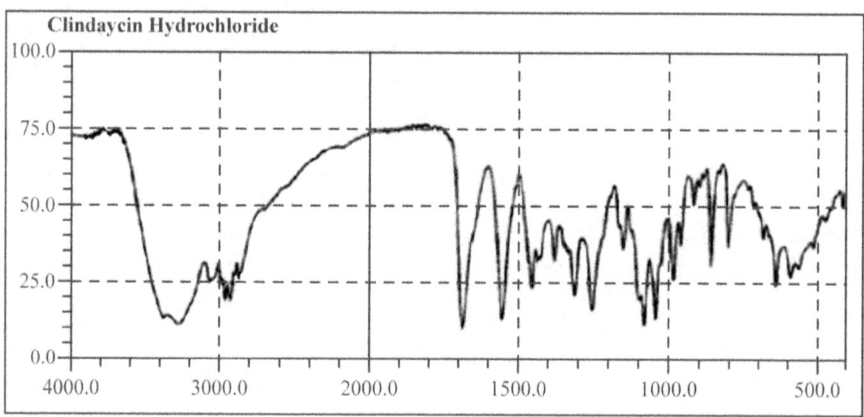

4. Ciprofloxacin hydrochloride

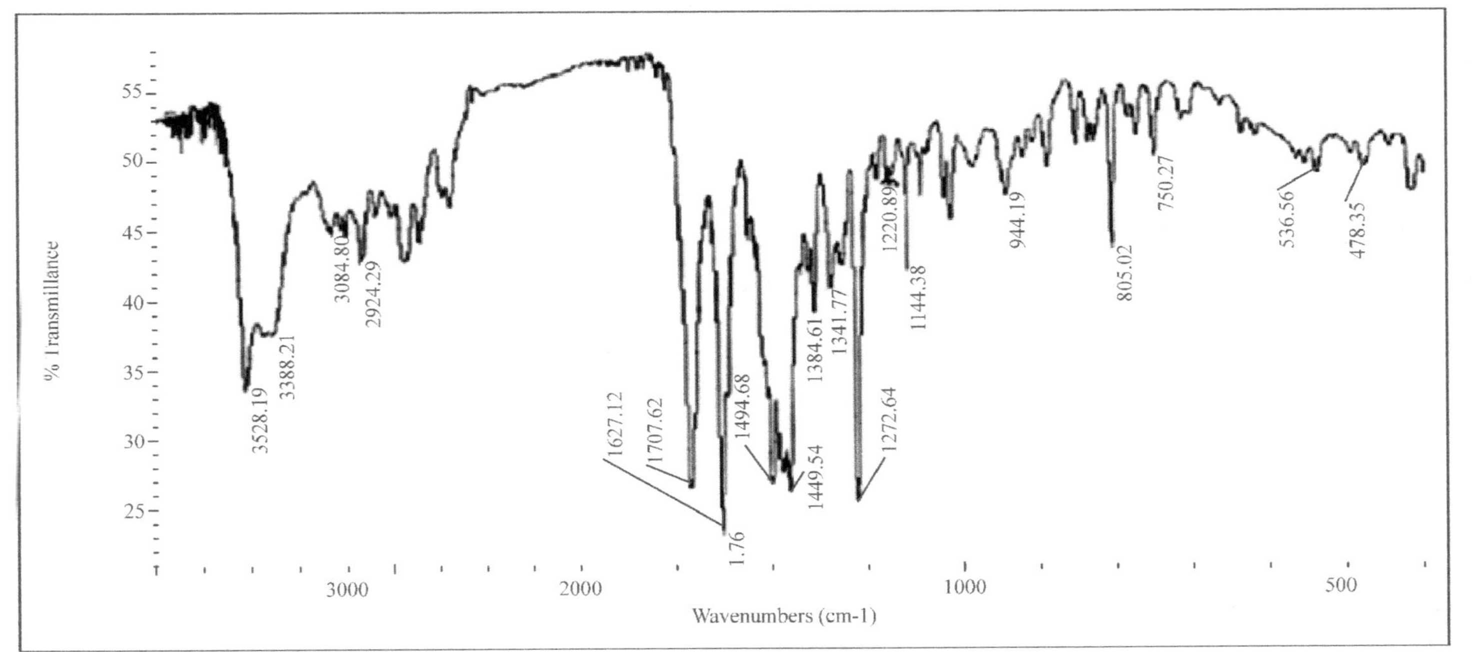

191

5. Caffeine

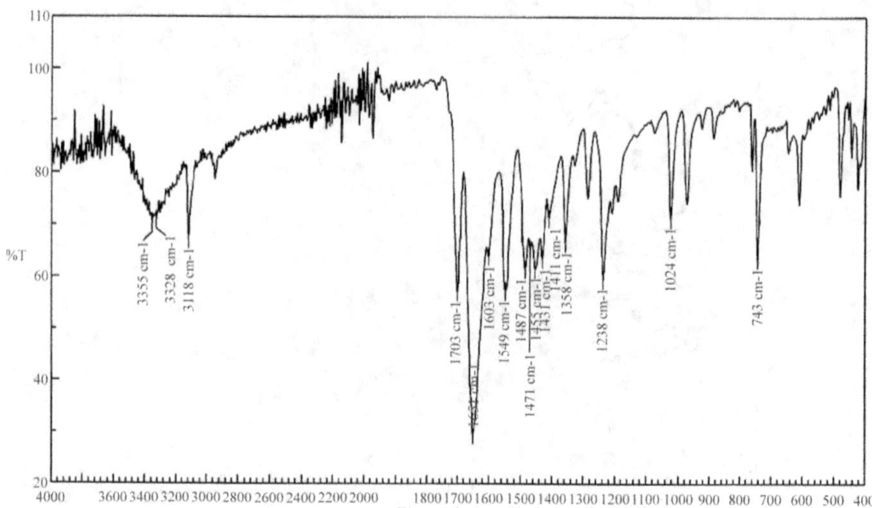

6. Acetic acid

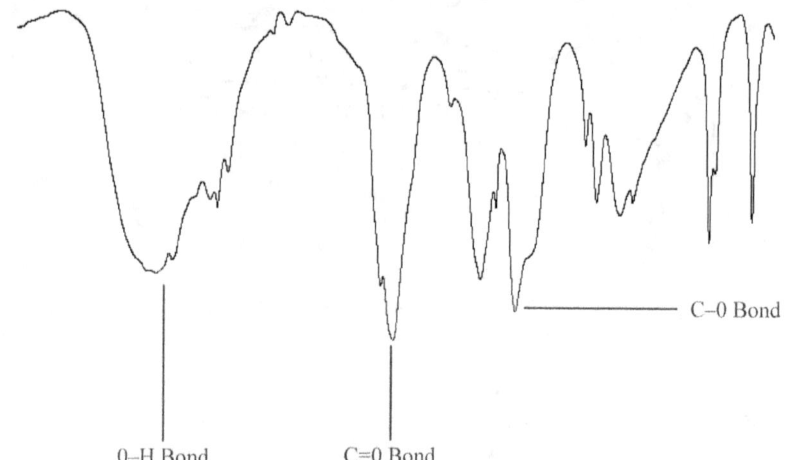

General Polymers Used in Pharmaceuticals

Polymer	Trade names	Available grades/ variations	Uses
Acrylic acid and butyl acrylate copolymer	ACRYSOL 644, ACUMER 1000, ACUMER 1110, Acusol 190, Acusol 420 N, Acusol 425 N, Acusol505N, Acusol573N	Acrylic/Acrylate Ester Copolymer, Acrylates Copolymer, Acrylic Acid Homopolymer, Acrylic/Maleic Copolymer etc.	Sensitive adhesive for transdermal patches
Alginic acid	Apyrosis, Natiriumalginaat	A7003, A2158, A2033, A0682 A1112 A71238	Oral and topical pharmaceutical products; thickening and suspending agent in a variety of pastes, creams, and gels, as well as a stabilizing agent for oil-in-water emulsions; binder and disintegrant
Carrageenan	Danagel™, Gelcarin®, Isagel™, Lactogel®, Lactarin™, SeaGel®, SeaKem®, and Viscarin®.	Refined (RC) Semirefined (SRC) Philippine natural *grade* (PNG), processed Eucheuma seaweed (PES) kappa, iota and labda	Modified release, viscosifier, stabilizing, thickening and gelling agent

Table *Contd...*

Polymer	Trade names	Available grades/ variations	Uses
Carboxy methyl cellulose	Klucel, Carmellose, Aqualon	10 mPa's to 100,000	Emulsion stabilizer, suspending agent and binder
Cellulose Acetate (2,3,6-Tri-O-acetyl cellulose; cellulose triacetate polymer; triacetylcellulose)	Clarifoil, Dexel, Tenite *Acetat*	CAB 398-3, 398-6, 398-10, 398-30	Matrix adsorbent beads, semipermeable membrane for dialysis, ultrafiltration and reverse osmosis and nano fibres
Cellulose acetate butyrate	Eastman CAB	CAB 171, 321, 381, 500, 531, 551, ranging from 1.1 Pa s and above	sustained release matrices and semipermeable membrane
Cellulose acetate phthalate	Aquateric	45.0–90.0 mPa s	Enteric coating Hydrocolloids
Chitosan	Poliglusam, Chitosan	High, medium, low	Cosmetics and controlled drug delivery applications, mucoadhesive dosage forms, rapid release dosage forms
Chloroprene and polychloropene	Duprene, polychloropene	……..	Synthesis of rubber, closures, Septum for injection, plungers for syringes, and valve components
Crosslinked sodium carboxy methyl cellulose	Ac-Di-Sol Croscarmelose	……..	disintegrant, superdisintegrant, carrier for dissolution enhancement, tablet additive
Cross Vinyl pyrrolidone	Crospovidone, Luvitec®K	……..	contact lenses, superdisintegrant and carrier for dissolution enhancement
Egg albumin	Egg Albumen powder, Egg protein powder, Egg white powder	Grade I, II, III, IV Flakes/ Powder	Binder, sustained release polymer
Ethyl Cellulose	Ashacel, Aquacoat®, Ethocel	3-385 mPa s	Aqueous coating system for sustained release applications
2-Ethylhexyl acrylate and butyl acrylate copolymer	ACM, Acrylamide	Old type, New type	Sensitive adhesive for transdermal patches
Gelatin	Gelatin, gelatin powder	acid processed, alkali processed	Plasma expander, sealant, capsules

Table *Contd…*

Polymer	Trade names	Available grades/ variations	Uses
Gum Tragacanth	Tragacanth gum, Tragacanth	powders, tears	binder, suspending agent, emulsifier, thickening agent, adhesive, stabilizer, drug (antidiarrheal, aphrodisiac, adaptogenic, laxative)
Polymetha-acrylates	Eudragits	ER, ER, ES, ERL, ERS, EE, ELD, ENED 50 - 200 mPa s	Glidant, plasticizer, sustained release, enteric coat
Hyaluronic acid	Hyaluronan	low molecular weight, high molecular weight	Reduction of scar tissue, cosmetics
Hydroxy ethyl cellulose	Natrosol, cellosize	3400-5000 cps	Bioadhesive, thickening agent, binder, slim coating and sustained release
Hydroxy propyl cellulose	Klucel	regular grind, fine grind Lactide-co-glycolide polymers	Binder, film coating and sustained release
Hydroxy propyl methyl cellulose	Hypromellose, hyprolose, cellulose	100 cps, K, M	antistatic, binder for tablet matrix and tablet coating, gelatin alternative as capsule material, stabilizer
Lactide-co-glycolide polymers	Lactide glycolide, Biodegmer, polyglactin, puralacto	ester end cup, acid end cup	Microparticle–nanoparticle for protein delivery
Methyl cellulose	Methocel, Methylcellulose	low, medium viscosity grade	binder, stabilizer, excipient, drug (bulk laxative)
Nitrile	Buna-N, Perbunan, Nipol, Krynac, Europrene®	sheet, crumb, powder, liquid	Disposable non-latex gloves, automotive transmission belts, hoses, O-rings, gaskets, oil seals, V belts, synthetic leather
Pectinic acid	Ingelheim, kinic acid, galacturonan	powder, crumbs	Drug delivery
Polyacetals	Delrin, ultraform, POM, acetal, Celcon, polyformaldehyde	H and C	sheets, tubes, rods

Table *Contd...*

195

Polymer	Trade names	Available grades/ variations	Uses
Poly (acrylic acid)	PAA, Carbomer	------	Cosmetic, pharmaceuticals, immobilization of cationic drugs, base for Carbopol polymers
Polyamides	Nylon, Ultramid	4-6, 6-10, 66	packaging, bulking and opacifying agent, textile industry
Polycarbonate	Merlon®, Macrolon, Lexan, Apex	Medium, high, low gloss, low gloss	Case for biomedical and pharmaceutical products
Polycyanoacrylate	Polyfix, Henke®, Super glue	methyl, ethyl, propyl	Biodegradable tissue adhesives in surgery, a drug carrier in nano- and microparticles
Poly (vinyl acetate)	Nikacol, alphamore, Vinnapas®		Binder for chewing gum, slow-*release* binders for fertilizer, photo printing plates, sponges for cosmetic
Polyethylene derivatives	polyethylene, polyethylene glycol, polypropylene	Poly (ethylene oxide) Poly (ethylene glycol)- Mw 1000 Polyethylene Polyethylene terephthalate	Coagulant, flocculent, very high molecular-weight up to a few millions, swelling agent Plasticizer, base for suppositories Transdermal patch backing for drug in adhesive design, wrap, packaging, containers Transdermal patch backing (when ethylene vinyl acetate copolymer is incompatible with the drug)
Polyisobutylene	Poly isobutene, oppanaol, Indopol, Panalane	PIB, PIB-1, PB-1	Pressure sensitive adhesives for transdermal delivery
Poly (isopropyl acrylamide) and poly (cyclopropyl methacrylamide)	------	------	Thermogelling
Polypropylene	Polyprene	------	Tight packaging heat shrinkable films, packaging and labelling

Table *Contd...*

Polymer	Trade names	Available grades/ variations	Uses
Polystyrene	Kalexate, polystyrate	homopolymer, block and random copolymer	Petri dishes and containers for cell culture
Poly (vinyl chloride)	Aurum, Bakelite,	Type I and II	Blood bag, hoses, and tubing
Polyurethane	Elastana, Lycra, Endoprene,	-----	Transdermal patch backing (soft, comfortable, moderate moisture transmission), blood pump, artificial heart, and vascular grafts, foam in biomedical and industrial products
Polyvinyl alcohol	Polyviol; Vinol; Alvyl; Alcotex; Covol; Gelvatol; Lemol; Mowiol; Mowiflex	Granular, powder	Water-soluble packaging, tablet binder, tablet coating
Polyacrylamide			Gel electrophoresis to separate proteins based on their molecular weights, coagulant, absorbent
Poly (vinyl pyrrolidone)	Prasol, polyvidone, povidone, copovidone	K-15, K-30, K-60, and K-90	Used to make betadine (iodine complex of PVP) with less toxicity than iodine, plasma replacement, tablet granulation, fining agent in wine industry
Silicones	-----	With talc and talc-less	Pacifier, therapeutic devices, implants, medical grade adhesive for transdermal delivery
Sodium starch glycolate	Explotab, Primojel, Vivastar P	A, B, C	Disintegrant, a suspending agent and as a gelling agent
Starch	Starch, Voluven	soluble, insoluble textile grade, food grade ionic, nonionic	Glidant, a diluent in tablets and capsules, a disintegrant in tablets and capsules, a tablet binder

Common surfactants with HLB Values and Use

Surfactants are typically ampiphilic molecules that contain both hydrophilic and lipophilic groups. The Hydrophile-Lipophile Balance (HLB) number is used as a measure of the ratio of these groups. It is a value between 0-60 defining the affinity of a surfactant for water or oil. HLB numbers are calculated for non-ionic surfactants, and these surfactants have numbers ranging from 0-20. HLB numbers >10 have an affinity for water (hydrophilic) and number <10 have an affinity of oil (lipophilic). Ionic surfactants have recently been assigned relative HLB values, allowing the range of numbers to extend to 60. In the formation of a stable emulsion, it is advisable to have a blend of two or more non-ionic surfactants rather than a single surfactant molecule. The HLB values of the surfactants are additive and the HLB value of the blend can be determined. For example, the HLB value of a 60% Tween 80 (HLB of 15) and 40 % Arlacel 80 (HLB of 4.3) is

Arlacel 80	$4.3 \times 0.4 = 1.7$
Tween 80	$15.0 \times 0.6 = 9.0$
	10.7

Example:

Sample Oil-in-Water lotion formula

- Mineral oil 8%
- Caprylic/capric triglyceride 2 %
- Isopropyl isostearate 2%
- Cetyl alcohol 4%
- Emulsifiers 4%
- Polyols 5%
- Water soluble active 1 %

- Water 74 %
- Perfume q.s.
- Preservative q.s.

Add up the oil phase ingredients

- Mineral oil 8%
- Caprylic/capric triglyceride 2%
- Isopropyl isostearate 2%
- Cetyl alcohol 4%

Total: 16%

Divide each by the total to get the contribution to the oil phase:

Mineral oil: 8 / 16 = 50%

Caprylic/capric triglyceride: – 2 / 16 = 12.5%

Isopropyl isostearate: – 2 / 16 = 12.5%

Cetyl alcohol – 4 / 16 = 25%

Multiply by the required HLB of the oil:

Mineral oil: 50.0% * 10.5 = 5.250

Caprylic/capric triglyceride: 12.5% * 5 = 0.625

Isopropyl isostearate: 12.5% * 11.5 = 1.437

Cetyl alcohol: 25.0% * 15.5 = 3.875

Add all values:

Total required HLB = 11.2

So, for this formulation, you would want to use a surfactant that has a value of approximately 11 to achieve the best emulsification.

HLB *values* are additive, so if the use of two different surfactants is desired, the HLB will be the weighted average of the HLB values for each product. For example, if you require an oil with an HLB of 11 in your formula, you could use 50% of a surfactant with an HLB of 12 (50% of 12 = 6) and 50% of a surfactant with HLB value of 10 (50% of 10 = 5). Total HLB = 6 + 5 = 11.

HLB system is not the absolute predictor of the behaviour of emulsion. Additional ingredients in the formula are not taken into account but may impact the stability of the emulsion. The HLB method also does not calculate exactly how much surfactant is needed, but a good starting point is 2 to 4%.

Below are the recommended HLB values of surfactants in various formulas:

- Mixing unlike oils together
  - Use surfactants with HLB of 1 to 3
- Making water-in-oil emulsions
  - Use surfactants with HLB of 4 to 6
- Wetting powders into oils
  - Use surfactants with HLB of 7 to 9
- Making self-emulsifying oils
  - Use surfactants with HLB of 7 to 10
- Making oil-in-water emulsions
  - Use surfactant blends with HLB of 8 to16
- Making detergent solutions
  - Use surfactants with HLB of 13 to 15
- For solubilizing oils (micro-emulsifying) into water
  - Use surfactant blends with HLBs of 13 to 18

Some oils require different HLB surfactants to form the most stable emulsion. The required HLB value for some of the most common oils used in pharmaceutical emulsions have been determined experimentally. Mixtures of these material will need a surfactant that matches the average HLB requirement of the oil components of the emulsion.

This table will help in selection of surfactant for Oil/Water and Water/Oil emulsions.

S. No.	Name	Description	HLB Value
1	Sodium lauryl sulfate	Sodium lauryl sulfate	40
2	PEG-PPG-PEG Pluronic® F-68 LF Pastille	Poly (ethylene glycol)-*block*-poly (propylene glycol)-*block*-poly (ethylene glycol) average M_n~8,400	□ 24
3	PEG-PPG-PEG Pluronic® L-35	Poly (ethylene glycol)-*block*-poly (propylene glycol)-*block*-poly (ethylene glycol) average M_n~1,900	18-23
4	Potassium oleate	Potassium oleate	20
5	Polyoxyethylene (100) stearyl ether	Brij® S 100 average M_n ~4,670	18
6	Sodium oleate	Sodium oleate	18
7	Polyoxyethylene sorbitan monolaurate	Tween 20	16.7
8	PPG-PEG-PPG Pluronic®10R5	Poly (propylene glycol)-*block*-poly (ethylene glycol)-*block*-poly (propylene glycol) average M_n~2,000	12-18

Table Contd...

S. No.	Name	Description	HLB Value
9	Polyoxyethylenesorbitan monopalmitate	TWEEN® 40 viscous liquid	15.6
10	Polyethylene glycol octadecyl ether Polyoxyethylene (20) stearyl ether	Brij® S20	15
11	Polyoxyethylene sorbitan monooleate	Tween 80	15
12	Polyethylene glycol sorbitan monostearate Polyoxyethylene sorbitan monostearate	TWEEN® 60 nonionic detergent	14.9
13	Polyoxyethylene sorbitan monolaurate	Tween 21	13.3
14	Polyethylene glycol octadecyl ether Polyoxyethylene (10) stearyl ether	Brij® S10 average M_n ~711	12
15	Triethanolamine oleate	Triethanolamine oleate	12
16	Polyoxyethylene sorbitan trioleate	Tween 85	11
17	Polyoxyethylene sorbitan tristearate	Tween 65	10.5
18	Sorbitan monolaurate	Span 20	8.6
19	Tetronic 701	Ethylenediamine tetrakis(propoxylate-*block*-ethoxylate) tetrol average M_n ~3,600	1-7
20	Tetronic 90R4	Ethylenediamine tetrakis(ethoxylate-*block*-propoxylate) tetrol average M_n~7,200	1-7
21	Span® 40	Sorbitan monopalmitate	6
22	Span 60	Sorbitan monostearate	4.8
23	Span 80	Sorbitan monooleate	4.3
24	Glyceryl monostearate	Glyceryl monostearate	3.8
25	Span 85	Sorbitan trioleate	1.8

Typical Release Kinetic Equations and Plots

1. Zero Order Release Kinetics

It is the process of constant drug release from dosage form and is independent of concentration of drug. The drug level in blood/ serum remains constant throughout delivery period from the dosage form.

$$Q = Q_0 + K_0 t$$

C_t is the amount of drug released at time t, C_0 is the initial concentration of drug at time $t = 0$,

K_0 is the zero-order rate constant.

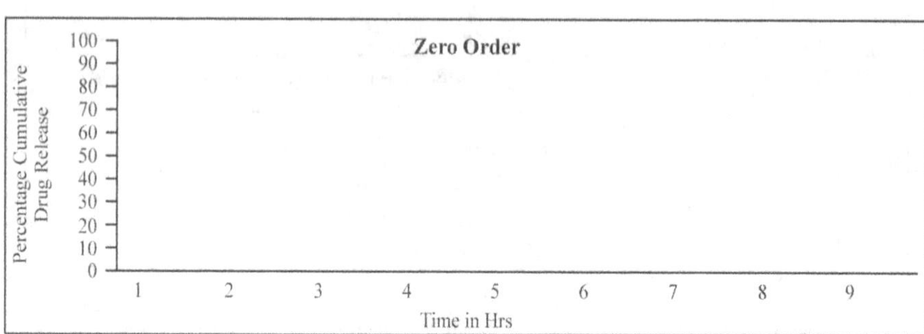

2. First Order Release Kinetics

The drug release is dependent on the concentration gradient between the static layer and the bulk liquid as seen mostly with dosage forms made using hydrophilic polymers or porous matrices.

$$DC/dt = - K_1 C$$

K_1 is the first order rate constant, expressed in time^{-1} or per hour.

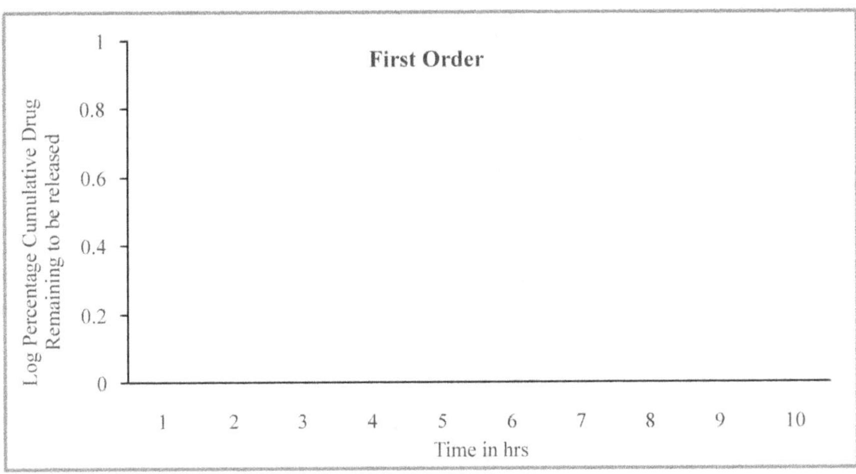

3. Higuchi Kinetics

The classical basic **Higuchi** equation is represented by. where Q is the cumulative amount of drug released in time t per unit area, C_O is the initial drug concentration, C_S is the drug solubility in the matrix and D is the diffusion coefficient of the drug molecule in the matrix. The zero-order rate describes the systems where the drug release rate is independent of its concentration. This explains why the drug diffuses at a comparatively slower rate as the distance for diffusion increases, which is referred to as square root **kinetics** (or **Higuchi's kinetics**).

$$Q = K_H \times t^{1/2}$$

where, K_H is the Higuchi dissolution constant, Q is the cumulative amount of drug released in time t per unit area, C_O is the initial drug concentration, C_S is the drug solubility in the matrix and D is the diffusion coefficient of the drug molecule in the matrix

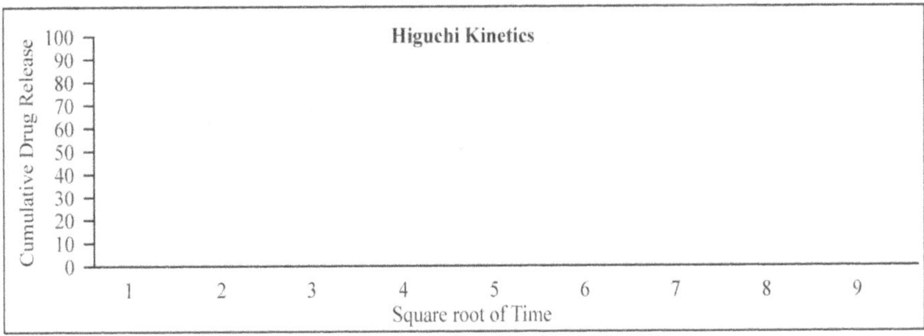

4. Korsemeyer Peppas Kinetics

To understand the dissolution mechanisms from the matrix, the release data were fitted using the well-known empirical equation proposed by Korsmeyer and Peppas. Korsmeyer and Peppas put forth a simple relationship which described the drug release from a polymeric system follow which type of dissolution. Mt/Mi is the fraction of drug released at time t over the total amount of drug released. To plot data according to **Korsmeyer-Peppas** model, data values only up to Mt/Mi=0.6 are used.

$$Mt/M\infty = K_{kp}t^n$$

Mt/M∞ is a fraction of drug released at time t,

M∞ is the amount of drug released after time ∞,

n is the diffusional exponent or drug release exponent,

K_{kp} is the Korsmeyer release rate constant.

To study release kinetics a graph is plotted between log cumulative % drug release log (M_t/M_∞) vs. log time (log t).

5. Hixon Crowell Equation

- The Hixson-Crowell cube root law describes the release from systems where there is a change in surface area and diameter of particles or tablets. Hence, particles of regular area are proportional to the cube root of its volume. From the above concept Hixson-Crowell established a relationship between drug release and time which can be represented by equation as

$$W_0^{1/3} - W_t^{1/3} = K_{HC}t$$

Where, W_0 is the initial amount of drug in the pharmaceutical dosage form (Amount of drug remaining at time 0).

- W_t is the remaining amount of drug in the pharmaceutical dosage form at time t; K_{HC} is the Hixson-Crowell constant describing surface volume relation.

- To study the release kinetics a graph is plotted between cube root of drug percentage remaining in matrix versus time.

Chapter 45

General Optimisation Techniques

The pharmaceutical formulations are prepared to provide optimum and best therapy to the patients with negligible and minimum side effects. It requires technicality and sound knowledge of different branches of pharmacy. Depending on the stakeholders in pharmacy profession it is required that the proper and required formulation is obtained in minimum time possible and in an economic way. As the processing of a new molecule from lab to market is an expensive and time consuming process, hence, use of automated systems and different analytical methods are used. But, getting a formulation requires trial and error leading to significant waste of chemicals, time and manpower.

For many years, pharmaceutical formulation scientists have used knowledge derived from individual experience to develop pharmaceutical dosage forms. The development of formulation and process are mostly based on intuitive and subjective judgement rather than a rational operation, therefore the whole process may or may not be optimal. Often formulation scientists are challenged with the problems of producing a final product which meets not only the requirements placed on it from a bioavailability standpoint, but also the practical mass production criteria of process and product reproducibility with limited time and funds. Trial and error approaches are inefficient and costly, and extrapolations made from them can be inaccurate. Stringent federal regulations, such as those promulgated by the Food and Drug Administration (FDA), require production process to be well-characterized and validated. In addition, during the development of a drug product for New Drug Application (NDA) submission, it is necessary to characterize the performance of the product during the process and to demonstrate that the final dosage form will behave in a predictable manner.

Optimization techniques are the research analytical tools for a problem which arc available to a researcher. These problems are related to pharmaceutical formulation, composition of the delivery system and process design. These involve mostly mathematical techniques in novel drug delivery systems. The classical optimization techniques are useful in finding the optimum solution or unconstrained maxima or minima of continuous and differentiable functions. These are analytical methods and make use of differential calculus in locating the optimum solution. The study of these classical techniques of optimization form a basis for developing most of the numerical techniques that have evolved into advanced techniques more suitable to today's practical problems. These methods assume that the function is differentiable twice with respect to the design variables and the derivatives are continuous. Three main types of problems can be handled by the classical optimization techniques: – single variable functions – multivariable functions with no constraints, – multivariable functions with both equality and inequality constraints. In problems with equality constraints the Lagrange multiplier method can be used.

Prominent examples include spectral clustering, matrix factorization, tensor analysis, and regularizations. These matrix-formulated optimization-centric methodologies are rapidly evolving into a popular research area for solving challenging data mining problems. These methods are amenable to vigorous analysis and benefit from the well-established knowledge in linear algebra, graph theory, and optimization accumulated through centuries. They are also simple to implement and easy to understand, in comparison with probabilistic, information-theoretic, and other methods. In addition, they are well-suited to parallel and distributed processing for solving large scale problems.

Optimization techniques are the research analytical tools for a problem which are available to a researcher. These problems are related to pharmaceutical formulation, composition of the delivery system and process design. These involve mostly mathematical techniques in novel drug delivery systems. In mathematics, optimization is the process of obtaining of maxima or minima. In most of the cases, Lagrangian method of optimization has been used for solving problems.

There are certain variables in optimization techniques regarding Pharmaceutical formulations:

These variables are of two types:

1. Independent variables
2. Dependent Variables

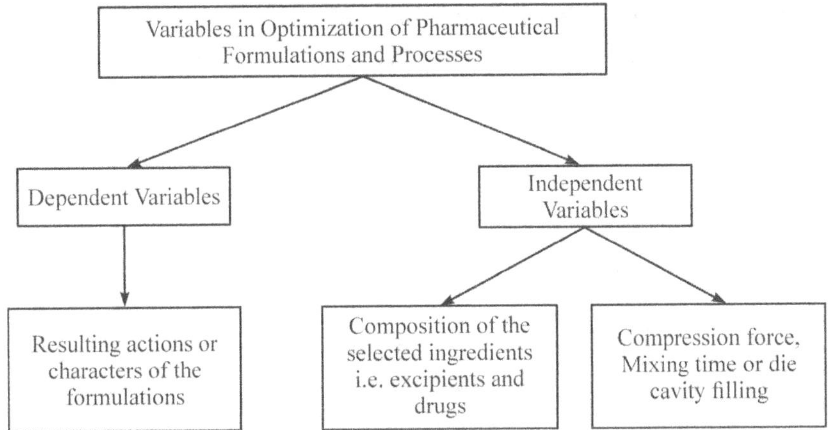

Optimization refers to obtaining resulting actions of our own interest by changing the independent variables one by one. Optimization is also sometimes referred to as multicriteria decision making.

There are two types of problem which are usually addressed in the optimization techniques:

1. Unconstrained
2. Constrained

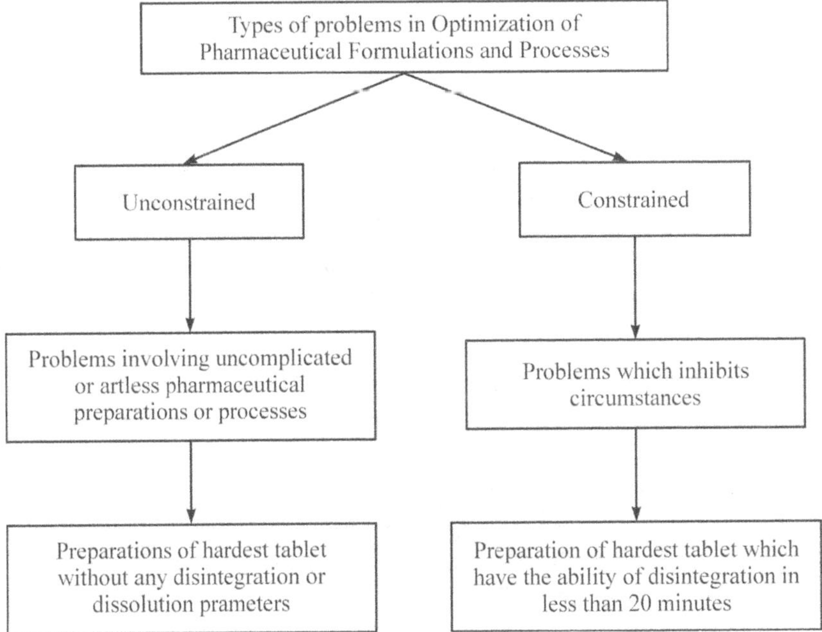

Mathematical form of Optimization Analysis

Classical optimization was analyzed by using graphs and calculus. In the case, when we use calculus Y is taken as a function of X.

$$Y = f(X)$$

When two independent variables are taken then

$$Y = f(X1, X2)$$

In the method of graphical representation, a simple graph of response along Y-axis is plotted along with an independent variable along X-axis showing a line with certain minimum or maximum values. When two independent variables are taken then the contour plots are drawn as shown below:

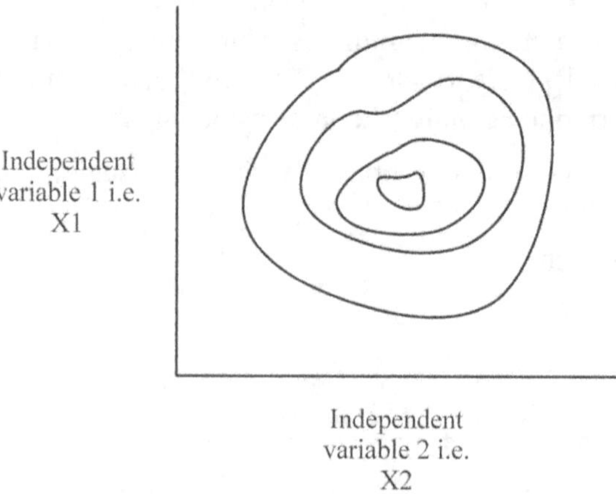

Here the contours are showing the resultant action/character i.e. response. (Contour represents the connecting point showing the peak level of something (such as response). Following type of response surface can be used for the analysis of dependent variable (Response or Resulting Action/Character) by changing the independent variables:

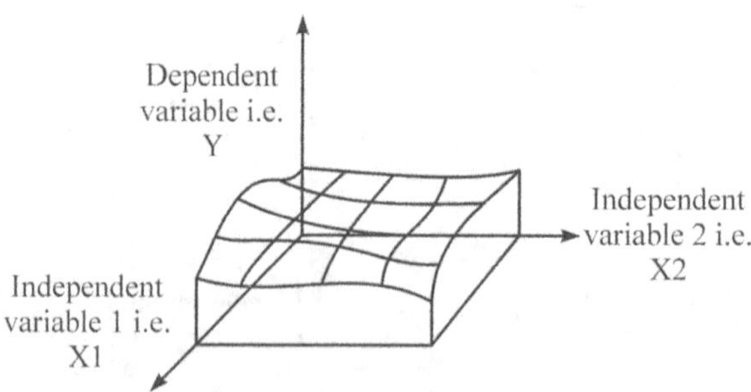

Response Surface in Optimization techniques of Pharmaceutical formulation and processing.

Methods for Optimization techniques

Several methods can be of use in Applied optimization:

1. Evolutionary operations
2. The Simplex methods
3. The Lagrangian Method
4. Search Method
5. Canonical Analysis

Forms of Optimization techniques:

There are three forms of systematic optimization techniques:

1. Sequential Optimization techniques.
2. Simultaneous Optimization techniques.
3. Combination of both.

1. Sequential Methods

This method is also referred to as the "Hill climbing method". As first of all a small number of experiments are done and further research will be done by using the increase or decrease of response. In this way a maximum or minimum will be reached i.e. an optimum solution.

2. Simultaneous Methods

This method involves the use of full range of experiments by an experimental design and the results are than used to fit in the mathematical model. And maximum or minimum response will then be found through this fitted model.

Artificial Neural Network (ANN) and Optimization of Pharmaceutical Formulations

ANN has been entered in pharmaceutical studies to forecast the relationship between the response variables and causal factors. This relationship is non-linear relationship. ANN is most successfully used in Multi-objective simultaneous optimization problem. (Takayama et al.) This problem arises when the favourable conditions of formulation for a single property may not be favourable for other characteristics. Radial basis functional network (RBFN) is proposed for multi-objective simultaneous optimization problem (Anand P et al.). RBFN is an ANN in which activation functions are radial basis functions (RBF). RBF is a function whose value depends only on the distance from the center or origin.

Applications

Through the optimization of the micro-encapsulation parameters such as shape of microcapsules, the strength of the microcapsule membranes and the membrane permeability of microcapsules now it is possible to develop more better forms of microcapsules for the treatment of diabetes and liver diseases.

Optimization techniques are also helpful in reducing the time of experimentation, study of pharmacokinetic parameters and High performance liquid chromatographic analysis.

One of the most important applications of Pharmaceutical optimization is found in the field of new drug discovery as the physicochemical and biological properties of a system can be improved by chemical modifications using Optimization techniques.

The application of an optimization technique consisting of statistically valid experimental design to pharmaceutical formulation development would provide an efficient and economical method to acquire the necessary information to understand the relationship between controllable (independent) variables and performance or quality (dependent) variables. The optimization process provides not only efficient use of resources, but also a method to obtain a mathematical model which can be used to characterize and optimize a formulation or process. Furthermore, by accurately defining the whole system, optimization techniques are a useful aid to process validation. The wet granulation process has been used as an alternative for high dose and poorly compressible active ingredients. It offers several advantages over other methods, for instance, it improves flowability, resistance to segregation and compression characteristics by increasing the particle size and cohesion.

A second advantage obtained when using optimization is the substantial time and cost savings due to the inherent efficiency of a rational experimental design. No theoretical model is required to be followed in advance of experimentation, curve fitting yields an empirical function. Subsequently, that function can be used to extrapolate results from those obtained at nodes in the experimental matrix to predict outcomes at points between the nodes, this allows one to draw tentative conclusions for hypothetical experiments, so that it may not be necessary to perform the actual experiment unless the prediction is favorable. One computer package called X-Stat (John Wiley and Sons) includes experimental design, data entry spreadsheets, curve fitting by various functions and contour plotting 1, 2 of results. Using contour plots, the effects of multiple factors may be viewed simultaneously, and conclusions drawn.

In general, the optimization process involves the following steps:

1. Analysis and define the problems

    (a) What are the objectives?

    (b) What is the nature of problem?

    (c) What is not known?

    (d) What is already known?

2. Based on previous knowledge and data, a preliminary choice can be made such as which process is to be adopted and which excipients are to be used.

3. Selection of a model, based on the results of the factor screening.

4. The experiments are designed accordingly and are executed.

5. The responses are analyzed for statistics by ANOVA. Test on lack of fit is done to get an empirical mathematical model for each individual response.

6. The responses are screened by using multiple criteria to get the values of independent variables. For example, restriction of hardness to 6-8 kg/cm^2 and disintegration time < 5 min for a tablet formulation to get the most probable values of the independent variables such as type of lubricants or their concentration, disintegrating agent, etc.

Experimental Designs

Experimental design is a statistical design that prescribes or advises a set of combination of variables. The number and layout of these design points within the experimental region depends on the number of effects that must be estimated. Depending on the number of factors, their levels, possible interactions and order of the model, various experimental designs are chosen. Each experiment can be represented as a point within the experimental domain. The point being defined by its co-ordinate (the value given to variables) in the space.

Factorial Design

Factorial designs were used in the 19th century by John Bennet Lawes and Joseph Henry Gilbert. Ronald Fisher argued in 1926 that "complex" designs (such as factorial designs) were more efficient than studying one factor at a time. A factorial design allows the effect of several factors and even interactions between them to be determined with the same number of trials as are necessary to determine any one of the effects by itself with the same degree. First, whenever we are interested in examining treatment variations, factorial designs should be strong candidates as the designs of choice. Second, factorial designs are efficient. Instead of conducting a series of independent studies we are effectively able to combine these studies into one. Finally, factorial designs are the only effective way to examine interaction effects.

(a) ***Full factorial design:*** It is an experimental design, which uses dimensional factor space at the corner of the design space. Factorial designs are used in experiments where the effects of different factors or conditions on choice for simultaneous determination of the effect of several factors and their interactions. The simplest factorial design is the 2 factorial designs, where two factors are considered each at two levels, leads to four experiments, which are situated in 2-dimensional factor space at the corners of a rectangle. If there are 3 factors, each at two levels, eight experiments are necessary which are situated at the corners of an orthogonal cube on a 3-dimensional space. The number of experiments is given by 2, where 'n' is the number of factors. If the number of factors and levels are large, then the number of experiments needed to complete a factorial design is large. To reduce the number of experiments, fractional factorial design can be used (i.e., ½ or ¼ of the original number of experiments with full factorial design). The fitting of an empirical polynomial equation to the experimental result facilitates the optimization procedure. The general polynomial equation is as follows: $Y = B0 + B1 X1 + B2 X2 + B3 X3 + B12 X1 X2 + B13X1 X3 + B23X2 X3$ —- Where Y is the response, X1, X2 , X3 are the levels (concentration) of the 1, 2, 3 factors and B1, B2 , B3 , B12, B13, B23, are the polynomial coefficients, B0 is the intercept (which represents the response when the level of all factors is low).

(b) ***Plackett-burman design:*** It is a fractional factorial design with $K = m*4$ experiment, for screening of (K-i) variables. Where K is the number of variables and m is the number of levels.

(c) ***Star design star design:*** is simply a 22 factorial design rotated over 45° angle in the space. A center point is usually added, which may be replicated to estimate experimental error, so there will be three levels for each factor where quadratic effect can be measured, but the interaction effect cannot be measured as in case of the full factorial design. In star design, 2k factorial designs are rotated over 45° in (k-i) direction in k-dimensional space with a replicated center point. k is the number of factors in the design. This results in 2k+R experiments, where R is the replicate of the center point.

(d) ***Central composite design:*** A better design that encompasses the advantages of factorial design or fractional factorial design or the star design, is the central composite design (CCD). This design is developed by Box and Wilson. It is composed of +2k Factorial design or Fractional factorial design.

2* k star design: This design enables the estimation of a full second-order model. The equation for two factors is given by $B0 + B1 X1 + B2 X2 + B12 X1X2 + B11 X12 + B22 X22$.

Box design: In central composite design each factor has five levels. If the number of factors increases, the number of experiments may become too high. The Box designs for three or more factors are economical alternative in which each factor is given three levels. The design is called an orthogonal balanced incomplete block design. It can be split into a set of incomplete blocks, which means that every effect is not estimated in every block, but every factor effect is measured as equal number of times with a balanced partition over the different blocks.

Doehiert hexagon or uniform shell design: Doehiert proposed uniform shell designs, starting with an equilateral triangle, mirrored in one side to a hexagon. The hexagon is expandable in 2- dimensional space by mirroring the center point in the outward sides. The equally spaced design points are uniformly distributed in concentric circles. It is also expandable in 3-dimension to concentric spherical shells. Due to the uniform distribution, models based on this design provide, a good basis for interpolation. A disadvantage may be that the number of levels is not same for all factors. The design may be started with one side of the hexagon parallel to the most important axis.

Mixture design: For mixtures of components (such as drugs and excipients in the formulation), special models have been derived, based on the mixture constraints. A fraction cannot be negative, and sum of the fractions of the components should be equal to one. An important property is that the number of coefficients to be estimated is reduced. The mixture constraint has consequences for the experimental designs. Factors cannot be chosen freely. In a two-component mixture, only one faction (variable) can be chosen, while in three component mixture only two fractions and so on. The remaining fraction completes the sum to one, which implies a dimension reduction. For k variable, the factor space can be represented geometrically by a (k-1) dimensional regular simplex, for two components a line, for three, a triangle and for four a tetrahedron.

Simplex lattice design: Simplex Lattice designs are used to explore the interior and the boundaries of the simplex. The number of factors determines its dimensions. The pattern of design points in the factor space and their number depend on the degree (the term of highest order) of the model that is postulated. The points are distributed orderly over the factor space, forming a lattice. The factors can be controlled accurately and precisely. The coefficients of model equations can be calculated easily.

Extreme-vertices design: It often occurs in formulation studies that the whole factor space is not accessible for experiment or that some areas are expected not to give useful responses. In an Extreme-Vertices design, observations are made at the corners of the bounded design space, at the middle of the edges and at the center of the design space. These can be used for the mixture composition as well as in combination with factorial designs.

Evolutionary methods: In the method the formulator makes a very small change in the formulation or process, but it makes so many times that he or she can determine statistical whether the product has improved. If it has been making another change in the same direction many times and notes. The results continues until further change do not improve the product. These methods are useful where there is a continue production. But due to the reasons like i) EVOP is not substitute to G.M.P ii) due to regulatory subject iii) because of the necessarily small changes utilized, it is not particularly suitable for lab.

D-Optimal: "D-Optimal" means that these designs maximize the information in the selected set of experimental runs with respect to a stated model. The D-Optimal design maximizes the determinant, of which is an overall measure of the information. Geometrically, this corresponds to maximizing the volume in a dimensional space. A D-Optimal design is suggested when:

- There is a linear constraint on the factor settings, reducing the experimental region to an irregular polyhedron. There are no classical designs that can well investigate an irregular region. A D-Optimal design is then the preferred choice as it makes efficient use of the entire experimental space.

- There are formulation factors, with lower and upper bounds, and possibly additional constraints, making the region an irregular polyhedron. There are qualitative factors, with more than two levels and there is no mixed level design available, or the mixed level design suggests too many runs to be acceptable.

- The objective is Response Surface Matter (RSM) and there are qualitative factors. The number of experimental runs affordable is smaller than the number of runs of any available classical design.

Chapter 46

Different Systems of Weights and Measures

Two types of measurement systems are distinguished historically: an evolutionary system, such as the British Imperial, which grew more or less haphazardly out of custom, and a planned system, such as the International System of Units (SI; Système Internationale d'Unités), in universal use by the world's scientific community and by most nations. There are two main systems for measuring distances and weight, the Imperial System of Measurement and the Metric System of Measurement. Most countries use the Metric System, which uses the measuring units such as meters and grams and adds prefixes like kilo, milli and centi to count orders of magnitude. In the United States, we use the older Imperial system, where things are measured in feet, inches and pounds.

- 1 mile equals 1.6 Kilometers.
- 1 yard is approximately 1 metre.
- 1 litre is about 1 American quart.
- 1 (UK) pint is about 500ml.
- 1 kilogram (kg) is about 2 pounds (lb).
- 1 inch is about 25 millimeters or 2.54 centimeters.
- A 3-foot measurement is almost exactly 1 meter.
- 1 Kilogram is just over 2 pounds.
- 1 pound is about 454 grams.
- For British visitors, 100 pounds = 7.14 stone.
- 0 degrees Celsius is equal to 32 degrees Fahrenheit. (The freezing point).
- 24 degrees Celsius is equal to 75 degrees Fahrenheit. (A very pleasant day).
- To convert Celsius (c) to Fahrenheit, use the formula $(c * 1.8) + 32$.

The English or Imperial System of Measurement

Length or distance

Lengths and distances are measured in inches, feet, yards and miles:

12 inches = 1 foot

3 feet = 1 yard

1760 yards = 1 mile

Fluid volume

Fluids are measured in fluid ounces, cups, pints, quarts and gallons.

The UK and American systems of fluid measurement are slightly different: the UK imperial system does not use cups, and the sizes are slightly different.

In the American system

8 fluid ounces (sometimes abbreviated to fl oz) = 1 cup

2 cups = 1 pint

2 pints = 1 quart

4 quarts = 1 gallon

In the English imperial system,

20 fluid ounces = 1 pint, and 'cups' are not used at all.

You're only likely to come across this as a problem in recipes, when it's usually clear whether you have an English or American recipe by the use of cups as a standard measure, and you can therefore amend your other measurements accordingly.

Weight

Weight is measured in ounces, pounds and tons

16 ounces (oz) = 1 pound (lb)

14 pounds = 1 stone (English imperial system only)

2,000 pounds = 1 ton

The Metric System

The metric system is much simpler. There are a series of *basic units*, one for each of distance, mass, and volume, and a series of prefixes to tell you what multiple of the basic unit is being used. The prefixes and what they mean are:

Prefix	Symbol	Meaning	Number
Giga-	G	One billion	1,000,000,000
Mega-	M	One million	1,000,000
Kilo-	K	One thousand	1,000
Deca-	D	Ten	10
(none)		One	1
Deci-	d	One tenth	0.1
Centi-	c	One hundredth	0.01
Milli-	m	One thousandth	0.001

British Imperial and U.S. Customary systems of weights and measures			
The U.S. uses avoirdupois units as the common system of measuring weight.			
Unit	Abbreviation or symbol	Equivalents in other units of same system	Metric equivalent
Weight			
Avoirdupois	avdp		
ton			
short ton		20 short hundredweight, or 2,000 pounds	0.907 metric ton
long ton		20 long hundredweight, or 2,240 pounds	1.016 metric tons
hundredweight	cwt		
short hundredweight		100 pounds, or 0.05 short ton	45.359 kilograms
long hundredweight		112 pounds, or 0.05 long ton	50.802 kilograms
pound	lb, lb avdp, or #	16 ounces, or 7,000 grains	0.454 kilogram
ounce	oz, or oz avdp	16 drams, 437.5 grains, or 0.0625 pound	28.350 grams
dram	dr, or dr avdp	27.344 grains, or 0.0625 ounce	1.772 grams
grain	gr	0.037 dram, or 0.002286 ounce	0.0648 gram
stone	st	0.14 short hundredweight, or 14 pounds	6.35 kilograms
Troy			
pound	lb t	12 ounces, 240 pennyweight, or 5,760 grains	0.373 kilogram
ounce	oz t	20 pennyweight, 480 grains, or 0.083 pound	31.103 grams
pennyweight	dwt, or pwt	24 grains, or 0.05 ounce	1.555 grams
grain	gr	0.042 pennyweight, or 0.002083 ounce	0.0648 gram

British Imperial and U.S. Customary systems of weights and measures			
The U.S. uses avoirdupois units as the common system of measuring weight.			
Unit	**Abbreviation or symbol**	**Equivalents in other units of same system**	**Metric equivalent**
Apothecaries'			
pound	lb ap	12 ounces, or 5,760 grains	0.373 kilogram
ounce	oz ap	8 drams, 480 grains, or 0.083 pound	31.103 grams
dram	dr ap	3 scruples, or 60 grains	3.888 grams
scruple	s ap	20 grains, or 0.333 dram	1.296 grams
grain	gr	0.05 scruple, 0.002083 ounce, or 0.0166 dram	0.0648 gram
Capacity			
U.S. liquid measures			
gallon	gal	4 quarts	3.785 litres
quart	qt	2 pints	0.946 litre
pint	pt	4 gills	0.473 litre
gill	gi	4 fluid ounces	118.294 millilitres
fluid ounce	fl oz	8 fluid drams	29.573 millilitres
fluid dram	fl dr	60 minims	3.697 millilitres
minim	min	$^1/_{60}$ fluid dram	0.061610 millilitre
U.S. dry measures			
bushel	bu	4 pecks	35.239 litres
peck	pk	8 quarts	8.810 litres
quart	qt	2 pints	1.101 litres
pint	pt	$^1/_2$ quart	0.551 litre
British liquid and dry measure			
bushel	bu	4 pecks	0.036 cubic metre
peck	pk	2 gallons	0.0091 cubic metre
gallon	gal	4 quarts	4.546 litres
quart	qt	2 pints	1.136 litres
pint	pt	4 gills	568.26 cubic centimetres
gill	gi	5 fluid ounces	142.066 cubic centimetres
fluid ounce	fl oz	8 fluid drams	28.412 cubic centimetres
fluid dram	fl dr	60 minims	3.5516 cubic centimetres
minim	min	$^1/_{60}$ fluid dram	0.059194 cubic centimetre

British Imperial and U.S. Customary systems of weights and measures			
The U.S. uses avoirdupois units as the common system of measuring weight.			
Unit	**Abbreviation or symbol**	**Equivalents in other units of same system**	**Metric equivalent**
Length			
nautical mile	nmi	6,076 feet, or 1.151 miles	1,852 metres
mile	mi	5,280 feet, 1,760 yards, or 320 rods	1.609 kilometres
furlong	fur	660 feet, 220 yards, or $^1/_8$ mile	201 metres
rod	rd	5.50 yards, or 16.5 feet	5.029 metres
fathom	fth	6 feet, or 72 inches	1.829 metres
yard	yd	3 feet, or 36 inches	0.9144 metre
foot	ft, or '	12 inches, or 0.333 yard	30.48 centimetres
inch	in, or "	0.083 foot, or 0.028 yard	2.54 centimetres
Area			
square mile	sq mi, or mi^2	640 acres, or 102,400 square rods	2.590 square kilometres
acre		4,840 square yards, or 43,560 square feet	0.405 hectare, or 4,047 square metres
square rod	sq rd, or rd^2	30.25 square yards, or 0.00625 acre	25.293 square metres
square yard	sq yd, or yd^2	1,296 square inches, or 9 square feet	0.836 square metre
square foot	sq ft, or ft^2	144 square inches, or 0.111 square yard	0.093 square metre
square inch	sq in, or in^2	0.0069 square foot, or 0.00077 square yard	6.452 square centimetres
Volume			
cubic yard	cu yd, or yd^3	27 cubic feet, or 46,656 cubic inches	0.765 cubic metre
cubic foot	cu ft, or ft^3	1,728 cubic inches, or 0.0370 cubic yard	0.028 cubic metre
cubic inch	cu in, or in^3	0.00058 cubic foot, or 0.000021 cubic yard	16.387 cubic centimetres
acre-foot	ac ft	43,560 cubic feet, or 1,613 cubic yards	1,233 cubic metres
board foot	bd ft	144 cubic inches, or $^1/_{12}$ cubic foot	2.36 litres
cord	cd	128 cubic feet	3.62 cubic metres

Drugs and their General Properties

Paracetamol

Structure

Chemical name: Acetaminophen; 4-Acetamidophenol; Paracetamol; 103-90-2; APAP; N-(4-Hydroxyphenyl) acetamide

Molecular formula: $C_8H_9NO_2$ or $HOC_6H_4NHCOCH_3$

Molecular weight: 151.165 g/mol

CAS number: 103-90-2

Physical description: Odorless white crystalline solid. Slightly bitter taste

Melting Point: 169-171

pKa: 9.38

Log P: 0.49

pH of saturated aqueous solution: 5.5-6.5

Dose:

Adults: 0.5-1g 4-6hrly (max 4 g.day-1)

Children older than one month: 20 mg.kg-1 6hrly (max 90 mg.kg-1.d-1)

Term neonates: 20 mg.kg-1 8hrly up to a maximum of 60 mg.kg-1.d-1).

Solubility: Paracetamol is poorly soluble in cold water, but more so in hot water. One part of paracetamol is soluble in 70 parts of water at room temperature, and 1 in 20 parts in boiling water. The aqueous solubility is elsewhere reported as 14.7 mg.ml-1 at 20°C, 14.3 mg.ml-1 at 25°C and 23.7 mg.ml-1 at 37°C. It is soluble in methanol, ethanol, dimethyl-formamide, ethylene dichloride, acetone and ethyl acetate. It is slightly soluble in ether and practically insoluble in petroleum ether, pentane and benzene

Pharmacokinetics

Absorption: Absolute bioavailability in the fasted fasting state ranges between 62%-89%. Peak concentrations are reached within 0.17 and 1.2 hours. The presence of food in the stomach decreases the absorption of paracetamol by increasing t_{max} and decreasing C_{max} values as it delays gastric emptying.

Distribution: The apparent volume of distribution of paracetamol is 0.69-1.36 L.kg-1. Plasma protein binding is 20%-25% at therapeutic doses. After overdosage, 20% - 50% of the drug may be protein bound. Paracetamol crosses the placenta and into breast milk, where 85% is bound to milk proteins.

Degradation

In vitro: Paracetamol degradation in vitro occurs through 2 pathways. It is either degraded by oxidation to quinone-imines or by hydrolysis of the amino group generating p-aminophenol. P-aminophenol is quickly degraded producing p-benzoquinoneimine. Deacetylation takes places both under acid and (much faster) basic conditions.

In vivo metabolism and elimination: *In vivo,* Paracetamol is metabolised primarily in the liver into non-toxic, inactive products via three metabolic pathways:

Glucuronidation is believed to account for 40% to two-thirds of the metabolism of paracetamol.

Sulfation (sulfate conjugation) may account for 20-40%.

N-hydroxylation and conjugation to glutathione accounts for less than 15%. The hepatic cytochrome P450 enzyme system (specifically CYPA2 and CYP2E1, and to a lesser extent CYP2D6) metabolizes paracetamol. A minor yet significant alkylating metabolite known as NAPQI (N-acetyl-p-benzo-quinoneimine) is formed. NAPQI is then irreversibly conjugated with the sulfhydryl groups of glutathione to form mercapturic acid conjugates and cysteine.

All three pathways yield final products that are inactive, non-toxic, and eventually excreted by the kidneys.

Elimination: Elimination is renally mediated but since only 5% of the drug is eliminated unchanged in the urine, patients with renal failure rarely have a prolonged drug effect. Plasma clearance is between 11.8-22.3 L.h-1. The elimination half-life is reported to be between 1.9 and 4.3 h.

UV λ_{max}: In ethanol- 250 nm

Nimesulide

Structure

Chemical name: Nimesulide; 51803-78-2; Mesulid; N-(4-Nitro-2-phenoxyphenyl) methanesulfonamide; Flogovital; Sulidene

Molecular formula: $C_{13}H_{12}N_2O_5S$

Molecular weight: 308.308 g/mol

CAS number: 51803-78-2

Physical description: It is a colorless to white, odorless powder with a bitter taste

Melting point: 143-144.5 °C

pKa: 6.5

Log P: 2.6

pH of saturated aqueous solution

Dose:

100-200 mg bid after food by oral route

For topical/cutaneous route-3%w/v gel or cream

Solubility-its water solubility is found to be 0.0182mg/ml

Pharmacokinetics

Nimesulide is absorbed rapidly following oral administration.

Nimesulide undergoes extensive biotransformation, mainly to 4-hydroxynimesulide (which also appears to be biologically active).

Food, gender, and advanced age have negligible effects on nimesulide pharmacokinetics.

Moderate renal impairment does not necessitate dosage adjustment, while in patients with severe renal impairment or hepatic impairment, Nimesulide is contraindicated.

Nimesulide has a relatively rapid onset of action, with meaningful reductions in pain and inflammation observed within 15 minutes from drug intake.

The therapeutic effects of Nimesulide are the result of its complex mode of action, which targets a number of key mediators of the inflammatory process such as: COX-2 mediated prostaglandins, free radicals, proteolytic enzymes, and histamine. Clinical evidence is available to support a particularly good profile in terms of gastrointestinal tolerability.

***The drug is now withdrawn from the market**

Biologic half-life- 1.8-4.7 hrs

Acceclofenac

Structure

Chemical name: Aceclofenac; 89796-99-6; Aceclofenaco; Aceclofenacum

Molecular formula: $C_{16}H_{13}Cl_2NO_4$

Molecular weight. 354.183 g/mol

CAS number- 89796-99-6

Physical description: It is white to almost white crystalline odorless powder having mild after bitter taste

Melting point: 149-153°C

pKa: 4.7

Log P: 3.98

Dose: 100 mg daily

Solubility: Aceclofenac is practically insoluble in water, freely soluble in acetone and in dimethyl formamide, and soluble in alcohol and in methanol.

Pharmacokinetics

Aceclofenac is rapidly and completely absorbed from the gastrointestinal tract and circulates mainly as unchanged drug following oral administration. The main route of elimination is via the urine where the elimination accounts for 70-80% of clearance of the drug. Approximately two thirds of the administered dose is excreted via the urine, mainly as glucuronidated and hydroxylated forms of aceclofenac. About 20% of the dose is excreted into feces. The volume of distribution is approximately 25 L. The mean clearance rate is approximately 5 L/h.

4'-hydroxyaceclofenac is the main metabolite detected in plasma however other minor metabolites include diclofenac, 5-hydroxy-aceclofenac, 5-hydroxydiclofenac, and 4'-hydroxydiclofenac [A19667]. It is probable that the metabolism of aceclofenac is mediated by CYP2C9. The mean plasma elimination half-life is approximately 4 hours.

UV λ_{max}: 276 nm

Ciprofloxacin hydrochloride

Structure

Chemical name: 1-cyclopropyl-6-fluoro-4-oxo-7-(piperazin-1-yl)-1,4-dihy-droquinoline-3-carboxylic acid hydrochloride

Molecular formula: $C_{17}H_{19}ClFN_3O_3$

Molecular weight: 367.805 g/mol

CAS number: 93107-08-5

Physical description: It is a Faint to light yellow crystalline powder.

Melting point: 225-257 °C

pKa: 6.09

Log P: 0.28

pH of 1% aqueous solution: 3.3 to 3.9

Dose

<18yrs: usually not recommended

Adults: 250 -750 mg as directed by the physician

Solubility: Soluble in dilute (0.1N) hydrochloric acid; practically insoluble in ethanol

In water, 30,000 mg/L at 20 °C

Pharmacokinetics

Ciprofloxacin for systemic administration is available as immediate-release tablets, extended-release tablets, an oral suspension, and as a solution for intravenous administration. When administered over one hour as an intravenous infusion, ciprofloxacin rapidly distributes into the tissues, with levels in some tissues exceeding those in the serum. Penetration into the central nervous system is relatively modest, with cerebrospinal fluid levels normally less than 10% of peak serum concentrations. The serum half-life of ciprofloxacin is about 4–6 hours, with 50-70% of an administered dose being excreted in the urine as unmetabolized drug. An additional 10% is excreted in urine as metabolites. Urinary excretion is virtually complete 24 hours after administration. Dose adjustment is required in the elderly and in those with renal impairment.

Ciprofloxacin is weakly bound to serum proteins (20-40%)

Ciprofloxacin is about 70% orally available when administered orally, so a slightly higher dose is needed to achieve the same exposure when switching from IV to oral administration

UV λ_{max}: 280 nm

Diclofenac sodium

Structure

Chemical name: Sodium diclofenac; Diclofenac sodium salt, sodium;2-[2-(2,6-dichloroanilino) phenyl] acetate

Molecular formula: $C_{14}H_{10}Cl_2NNaO_2$

Molecular weight: 318.129 g/mol

CAS number: **15307-79-6**

Physical description: It is white to off white in color, odorless, crystalline and slightly hygroscopic in nature.

Melting point: 288-290°C

pKa: 4.15

Log P: 4.51

pH of saturated aqueous solution-

Dose: 50-75 mg orally 2-3 times a day

Solubility: Sodium salt is soluble in water, sodium hydroxide, alcohol, acetone and phosphate buffer. It is insoluble in acid, cyclohexane and chloroform. The water solubility is 50mg/mL.

Pharmacokinetics

Diclofenac sodium after oral administration is well absorbed and with a plasma half-life of 1-3 hrs. Highest concentrations are found in bile, liver and kidney followed by blood, heart and lungs. Like other NSAIDs, it is also bond to plasma proteins (more than 99.5%) especially to albumin.

UV λ_{max}: 276 nm

Experiment 48

Standard Operating Procedures (SOPs)

Object

Standard operating procedures of various equipment and techniques.

1. SOP for Good Laboratory Practice (GLP)

1. While performing any analysis always follow respective standard operating procedure.
2. Use only pure (AR / GR grade) material for standardization.
3. Use calibrated volumetric glassware only, when accurate dilutions are required.
4. Ensure that the temperature during dilution, at the time of volumetric measurement and standardization is maintained i.e., at about 25°C.
5. Rinse the burette or other vessel used to collect the volumetric solution with the solution to be standardized.
6. While dilution always add concentrated acid slowly to the water, and never add water to acid.
7. Handle the chemicals and solvents in a way to avoid spillage on the working bench and the floor.
8. In case of any spillage immediately clean the affected area, according the type of spillage.
9. Wear a full-seal goggles and safety mask while handling concentrated acids and bases.
10. Never try and adjust the pH of a solution in a narrow-neck container. Always use a beaker.
11. Never stick a spatula in to a container of a solid reagent. Always roll the container to deliver the reagent in a controlled manner to the receiving beaker.

12. Never return unused reagent to the reagent container. Contamination of the whole reagent supply is more costly than the small amount of reagent discarded.

13. Use water for injection, unless otherwise specified, for preparation and standardization of solution.

14. Use water for injection for preparation of buffer solution, indicator solution, standard solution unless otherwise specified.

15. Standardize the volumetric solution with that method only which is used for endpoint determination.

16. Store the light sensitive solution in the light resistant (amber coloured) containers only.

17. Label all the reagents for Name, strength, prepared by & on and shelf life.

18. While performing titration in case of colourless solutions in the burette, consider the lower meniscus as the reading. In case of coloured solutions consider upper meniscus.

19. Always fill burette taking it away from the stand in to the hand and using a glass funnel. Adjust the reading to zero before starting titration.

20. Use approximately 0.1 mL of indicator, during titration or standardization, unless otherwise specified.

21. Never use broken glass-wares and in case of iodometric titration use iodine flask.

22. Store toxic and flammable chemicals in the separate area under lock and key.

23. Store all the reference standards and stock of working standards in their Specified area.

24. Working standards in use are to be stored in the desiccator provided. And the bottles are sealed immediately after their use.

25. Never leave any chemical reaction taking place on the gas i.e. boiling, distillation, refluxing unattended.

26. While boiling anything, keep the container opened, if not refluxing.

27. Check the LPG cylinder and pressure tubing for any damage or leakage; change the tubing if damage or leakage is found.

28. Always close LPG valve first and then put off the compressor while working with them, there is a chance of explosion when compressor is closed first.

29. Always keep the burner OFF while mopping the LAF bench.

30. After completion of any microbiological work, put on the UV light.

31. Never look directly into the UV light.

32. For analysis always use calibrated instruments.

33. If instrument / equipment found damaged, do not use it and consult Q. C. Manager / executive to get it repaired or changed.

34. While cleaning any electrode of either pH meter or conductivity meter, clean them with water for injection and wipe off with the help of a tissue paper gently.

35. Never rub the electrode and keep all the electrodes dipped constantly on the water for injection.

2. SOP for Glassware Washing

Preparation of cleaning solutions- For the cleaning of glassware those are used for chemical analysis special precautions will take place to avoid any chemical residue in glassware, which may later interfere with the results of chemical analysis. Following cleaning solutions were used for cleaning of glassware:

- 0.5% Labolene
- 2% Liquid soap solution
- 0.5% Labolene

1. Cleaning of glassware, which has contained hazardous materials, must be solely undertaken by experienced personnel.

2. Most new glassware is slightly alkaline in reaction. For precision chemical tests, new glassware should be soaked several hours in acid water (1% solution hydrochloric acid or nitric acid) before washing.

3. Wash glassware as quickly as possible after use if it is not possible then the articles should be allowed to soak in water.

4. For cleaning of glassware such as bottles, flasks, beakers, test tubes, etc use 0.5% Labolene. For better results use hot water.

5. For general cleaning 2% liquid soap solution may also be used when Labolene are not available.

6. During the washing all parts of the article should be thoroughly scrubbed with a brush selected for the shape and size of the glassware. Brushes should always be in good condition to avoid any abrasion of the glassware.

   Special types of precipitate material may require removal with nitric acid, aqua regia or fuming sulphuric acid. These are very corrosive substances and should be used only when required.

7. Before cleaning of glassware remove the labelling of marker pen with the help of IPA or acetone. For plastic ware do not use acetone for removing marker pen labelling.

8. It is required that all soap detergents and other cleaning fluids be removed from glassware before use. This is especially important with detergents, slight traces of which will interfere with serological and culture reactions. After cleaning, thoroughly rinse with tap water ensuring that containers are partly filled with water, shaken and emptied several times. Finally rinse with purified water.

9. After cleaning dry the glassware in Hot air oven at 60 °C temperature ± 5 °C.

10. Always protect clean glassware from dust by use of temporary closures or by placing in a dust free cabinet.

3. SOP for the Process of Sterilization and Disinfection

Principle: Hot air oven is used for dry heat sterilization. Material to be sterilized is completely dried and hence to make it free from live spore, a temperature in the range of 165-170°C should be used. Usually 165°C for a period of two hours is sufficient for the desired effect.

Operating procedure

1. Set the desired temperature and adjust heater switch to a suitable position.

2. Set the desired temperature in the digital temperature controller.

3. Push red push switch, hold and rotate in anticlockwise or clockwise directions to increase or decrease the set temperatures.

4. Release the red push switch to start relay indicated by the light emission devices (LED).

5. Allow the oven to achieve the set temperature upon which the LED is put off indicating relay cut off and the desired/set temperature is achieved.

6. After the operation is over switch off the mains switch and the electrical supply.

Precaution and maintenance

1. Do not open door immediately after the lapse of proposed time. Allow it to cool up to 60°C.

2. Do not keep material which will get distorted at the operational temperature.

3.   Do not keep moist articles. Dry it prior to loading in sterilizer.

4.   Keep the ventilating side open till temperature reaches 80°C, to remove residual moisture.

5.   SOP for Magnetic Stirrer.

Principle: Magnetic propeller rotates teflon bar and facilitate stirring.

Operating procedure

1.   Connect to mains and switch on.

2.   Place the beaker / vessel containing the solution to be stirred on the hot plate of magnetic stirrer. Put Teflon bar (magnet) in the beaker.

3.   Switch on the instrument.

4.   Adjust heating rate using 'heat' knob. Adjust rotation speed using knob.

5.   Turn off the switch when stirring work is completed.

Precaution and maintenance

1.   Remove the plug from power point when instrument is not in use.

2.   Avoid spillage of liquid over platform. Clean it properly after use.

4. SOP for Centrifuge

Principle: A centrifuge driven by an electric motor that puts an object in rotation around a fixed axis, applying a force perpendicular to the axis. The centrifuge works using the sedimentation principle, where the centripetal acceleration causes more dense substances to separate out along the radial direction (the bottom of the tube).

Operating procedure

1.   Open the lid.

2.   Take clean tubes and fill the same as per the recommended filling capacity.

3.   When fitting the loaded bucket tubes to the rotor always distribute them   asymmetrically around the rotor axis to avoid destructive vibration.

4.   Place all the buckets in the rotor even if these are not needed for centrifuge.

5.   Before placing the reducing rubber adaptors in the metal tubes, remove the profiled rubber cushions.

6.   Close the centrifuge lids.

7. Switch on the mains switch of the machine. The timer will start blinking indicating 00.

8. In this mode the centrifuge can be started and used by pressing the timer i.e. on

9. For using the timer in the time mode press the set time switch. It will show 00 minutes.

10. The desired time can now be selected by pressing set time switch again.

11. The centrifuge is now ready to operate in time mode.

Precaution and maintenance

1. Use only, polyamide tubes in the angle rotor heads as the glass tubes will break as high centrifuge forces are attained by the angle rotors.

2. Do not open the lid while the instrument is in operation.

3. Check the stirrer for any mechanical/electrical faults and breakdown.

4. After about 1000 hours of operation or about 6 months the bearing of the motor should be lubricated to avoid breakdown.

Calibration: Ensure that all connections of instrument are proper. Operate the instrument as per the operating instructions. Use duly calibrated tachometer, digital thermometer and stop watch during calibration of the equipment.

5. SOP for Incubator

Principle: Microbiology incubators are designed to promote the growth of microorganisms by maintaining a constant temperature within a narrow range.

Operating procedure

1. The display toggles, light emission device (LED) indicator glows and displays the chamber temperature. Adjust required temperature with the help of thermostatic control knob.

2. Keep the 'set' knob pressed and adjust temperature using the 'coarse' knob, and fine tune the temperature using 'fine' knob.

3. After setting the desired temperature release the red push switch the relay starts and is indicated by the light emission devices. Allow the temperature to rise to set temperature and stabilize. Open the door of the instrument & load the samples in the plates/ test accessories.

4. Observe the temperature by calibrated thermometer dipped in glycerol kept inside the incubator and record the observations.

Precaution and maintenance

1. Install the unit at least one foot away from the wall on the rear.
2. Ensure that the glass door is always closed before the outer door.

6. SOP for Analytical Balance

Principle: The principle of analytical balance is a simple lever with weights on one side of the fulcrum that balance the weight of the unknown object in the pan.

Operating procedure

1. Rotate the weighing knob clockwise. Open slide door and put butter paper on pan.
2. Then place weight on left hand pan, and sample on right hand pan.
3. Close the slide door and rotate weighing knob anticlockwise. Check position of central needle.
4. Rotate weighing knob clockwise, and add or withdraw the sample/weight, as required and bring central needle at the central point of scale.
5. Open slide door, take out sample, clean pan properly after use and close the slide doors.

Performance check

After the auto calibration, put 1, 2, 5, 10 and 20 mg weights individually. The measurement shall be within the 0.1% of actual mass value of the individual weight as given in the performance check log.

Measurement uncertainty check

The measurement of uncertainty shall be carried out by using 10 mg weight. Put the external weight of 10 mg on the pan and note the 10 measurements. Calculate the measurement of uncertainty.

Measurement of uncertainty shall be not more than 0.001.

Calibration frequency: It shall be performed daily, after any maintenance, after the relocation and after the power failure of the balance. Before calibration, make sure that the level bubble is in the center of the indicator and if internal calibration facility is available in the balance then it shall also be performed daily before performance check of the balance.

Precautions & maintenance

1. Do not shift the balance once positioned.

2. Close the glass doors on the sides and top before recording the weights.

3. After completion of weighing keep the inside area clean.

7. SOP for Dispensing Balance

Principle: The principle of dispensing balance is a simple lever with weights on one side of the fulcrum that balance the weight of the unknown object in the pan.

Operating procedure

1. Put butter paper on both pan of same size.

2. Place weight on left hand pan, and sample on right hand pan.

3. Lift the weighing lever anticlockwise, and see the position of central needle.

4. Add or withdraw the sample/weight, as required and bring central needle at the central point of scale.

5. Take the sample out clean the pan properly after use and close the slide doors.

Precautions & maintenance

1. Do not shift the balance once positioned.

2. After completion of weighing keep the inside area clean.

8. SOP for Microscope

Principle: A general biological microscope mainly consists of an objective lens, ocular lens, lens tube, stage, and reflector. An object placed on the stage is magnified through the objective lens. When the target is focused, a magnified image can be observed through the ocular lens.

Operating procedure

1. Clean the exposed optical surfaces with a soft cotton cloth.

2. Plug the electrical cord into an electrical supply.

3. Bring the light intensity regulator to the lowest level.

4. Switch on the power supply.

5. Adjust the observation head to a convenient working position.

6. Rotate the nose piece until the lowest power objective is in the viewing position.

7. The lower is the power of the objective the greater is the field of view.

8. Take down the stage to a fairly low position with the help of a coarse focus knob.

9. Make sure that the stage surface is free from dust, grit or any other material that might interfere in the specimen movement across the surface of the stage.

10. Position the specimen area of the slide over the centre of the stage aperture.

11. Use the stage control knob to move the specimen slide to the desired position.

12. Looking through the observation head, raise the stage by adjusting the coarse focus knob until an image appears.

13. Focus as sharply as possible with the coarse focus adjustment knob.

14. Adjust the fine focus knob to sharpen the image in the center of the field of view.

15. Look at the image and adjust the diaphragm aperture to obtain the clearest possible image. (Clarity of image depends upon the size of the aperture ; as the aperture becomes smaller the contrast and the depth of the focus increases but resolution power decreases).

Precaution and maintenance

1. Never touch the lenses with fingers.
2. Always clean the lens with neat cloth.
3. Do not handle the microscope with its lens body.

9. SOP for Water Bath

Principle: Vapors of water filled in instrument provides mild and indirect heating.

Operating procedure

1. Switch on the power supply.
2. Check and maintain the water level in water bath.
3. Securely cover the lids of stations of water bath.
4. Switch on the mains switch of water bath.
5. Set the temperature of water bath by pushing the "press to set" switch and by "set" and "fine" knobs.
6. Place the vessels in stations of water bath.
7. Switch off the mains switch of when work is completed.
8. Switch off the power supply.

Precaution and maintenance

1. Always maintain water level as if water is not sufficient instrument may be damage.
2. Remove the plug from power point when instrument is not is use.
3. Clean the assembly after use.

10. SOP for Dissolution Test Apparatus

Principle: The main operating principle for dissolution apparatus (paddle/basket) is to provide precise stirring and mixing at 37 °C.

Operating procedure

1. When the power is switched on the timer and temperature shows digital value.
2. Set the temperature to 37°C by using set temp and enter key.
3. Set the timer by using clock and enter key.
4. Set the interval for sampling by using set interval and enter key.
5. Fill the tank with purified water and adjust the temperature between 37 ± 1 °C.
6. Place the test sample in the test vessel.
7. Start the apparatus by using the start test key.
8. After sometime collect the samples with the help of sampling cannulas at regular time intervals when the buzzer sounds.
9. After complete dissolution of test sample, Press the stop test key from the front panel.
10. Discard the solution and rinse the vessel.
11. Switch off the main switch and heater switch of dissolution apparatus.

Precaution and maintenance

1. Remove the water of water bath after completion of work.
2. Properly clean the instrument after completion of work.
3. Routinely check instrument for any damage and corrosion.

11. SOP for Heating Mantle

Principle: Heating can be achieved by heating of coil of the instrument.

Operating procedure

1. Connect to mains and switch on the mains switch.
2. Set required temperature using temperature regulator knob.

3. After the temperature reached to the required level place the vessel in pit of the heating mantle.

4. Turn off the switch when work is completed.

Precaution and maintenance

1. Switch off the instrument if any unusual smell of burning is observed.

2. Do not spread any liquid in coil of the apparatus.

12. SOP for Mechanical Stirrer

Principle: Mechanical shaking by the wrist type movement of the apparatus resulting in the mixing of ingredients.

Operating procedure

1. Clamp the containers [vials/ ampoules] tightly.

2. Set the knob at minimum and then switch on the main switch.

3. Set the shaking speed using knob.

4. Switch off the mains after completion of work.

Precaution and maintenance

1. Clamp glasswares properly.

2. Cover the instrument after completion of work.

13. SOP for Mechanical Shaker

Principle: Mechanical shaking by the wrist type movement of the apparatus resulting in the mixing of ingredients.

Operating procedure

1. Clamp the containers [vials/ ampoules] tightly.

2. Set the knob at minimum and then switch on the main switch.

3. Set the shaking speed using knob.

4. Switch off the mains after completion of work.

Precaution and maintenance

1. Clamp glasswares properly.

2. Cover the instrument after completion of work.

14. SOP for Mechanical Shaker

Principle: Mechanical shaking by the wrist type movement of the apparatus resulting in the mixing of ingredients.

Operating procedure

1. Clamp the containers [vials/ ampoules] tightly.

2. Set the knob at minimum and then switch on the main switch.

3. Set the shaking speed using knob.

4. Switch off the mains after completion of work.

Precaution and maintenance

1. Clamp glasswares properly.

2. Cover the instrument after completion of work.

15. SOP for Melting Point Apparatus

Principle: Substances melt on heating.

Operating procedure

1. Put the capillary tube filled with sample and thermometer in respective holes.

2. Switch on the instrument.

3. Switch on the heater and lamp.

4. Note the melting range.

5. Switch off the mains after completion of work.

Precaution and maintenance

1. Ensure the temperature of instrument is normal before the use.

2. Use only calibrated thermometer.

3. Calibrate the instrument once in a month.

16. SOP for pH Meter

Principle: A pH meter is essentially a voltmeter with high input impedance which measures the voltage of an electrode sensitive to the hydrogen ion concentration, relative to another electrode which exhibits a constant voltage.

Operating procedure

1. Pull up the electrode and remove the beaker of distill water.

2. Keep a beaker / container below the electrode. Wash the electrode with distilled water.

3. Remove the container and blot dry the electrode with tissue paper or a suitable soaking device.

4. Dip the electrode in the solution for which the pH is to be measured, press the on/off keypad.

5. Note the pH reading from the display screen after it is stable for at least 30 sec and ready appears on the screen.

6. Turn the on /off key off, dip the electrode in the beaker containing distill water.

17. SOP for Electronic Balance

Principle: The electronic balance has a load cell pressure transducer. It converts the weight in to a proportional electrical signal. The sensing resistance in the load cell forms a Wheatstone bridge.

Operating procedure

1. Ensure that the balance is properly connected to the power supply.
2. Check the level with the spirit level. Switch on the main switch.
3. Close the glass windows properly. Press the on/off power switch.
4. Internal calibration begins. Upon completion of calibration the screen shows off.
5. Press the power switch, the screen displays 0.0000 and ready for weighing.
6. Weigh the samples using a fresh butter paper

Frequency

Internal calibration and accuracy = Daily, Precision: Once in a month

Precaution and maintenance

1. Switch off the electric supply if it is on.
2. Don't use wet cloth for cleaning.
3. Remove the plug from the socket.
4. Doesn't use wet cleaning agents on the electrical points/knobs/ wires.
5. Clean the balance without disturbing the position of the same.

Principle: The electronic balance has a load cell pressure transducer. It converts the weight in to a proportional electrical signal. The sensing resistance in the load cell forms a Wheatstone bridge.

Operating procedure

1. Ensure that the balance is properly connected to the power supply.
2. Check the level with the spirit level. Switch on the main switch.
3. Close the glass windows properly. Press the on/off power switch.
4. Internal calibration begins. Upon completion of calibration the screen shows off.
5. Press the power switch, the screen displays 0.0000 and ready for weighing.
6. Weigh the samples using a fresh butter paper.

Frequency:

Internal calibration and accuracy = Daily, Precision: Once in a month.

Precaution and maintenance

1. Switch off the electric supply if it is on.
2. Don't use wet cloth for cleaning.
3. Remove the plug from the socket.
4. Doesn't use wet cleaning agents on the electrical points/knobs/ wires.
5. Clean the balance without disturbing the position of the same.

18. SOP for Rotamantle

Principle: Based on the principles of thermodynamics conduction, insulation prevents glassware from any excessive temperature gradients while rotating.

Operating procedure

1. Put the properly clamped flask over mantle.
2. Switch on the rotamantle.
3. Set temperature by turning the knob.
4. Set the rotation of stirrer using the knob.
5. Switch of the mantle after completion of work.
6. Clean it properly.

Precaution and maintenance

1. Avoid spillage of liquid on mantle.
2. Switch off the mantle, if liquid goes inside the instrument.
3. Always keep mantle properly cleaned.

19. SOP for Deep Freezer

Principle: Exchange of heat with product, gradually brings it to the desired temperature where its enzymatic and chemical processes ceases and degradation is prevented.

Operating procedure

1. Connect the unit to properly rated power point.
2. Place the shelves at the required height and loaded the freezer with sample.
3. Press the main switch to on position and see that the lamp is illuminated.

4. Set the required temperature by pressing push and then rotating the set knob.

5. Depending on the temperature required cooling will start till the set temperature is reached.

Precaution and maintenance

1. Connect the unit to the correct electrical supply line of 230 volts 50 Hz.

2. Single phase should have at least 15 Amps Current Carriage capacity.

3. Use of good quality voltage stabilizer is must to protect against fluctuating power and load shedding conditions.

4. Time delay for the system is 200 seconds.

5. Clean the chamber and shelves at regular intervals and allow the Deep Freezer to defrost every week by switching off the unit for at least for 2 hours.

20. SOP for Environmental Test Chamber

Principle: Environmental test chamber is based on the microprocessor controlled   temperature and RH condition.

Operating procedure

1. Connect to mains and switch on the mains switch.

2. If the unit was in stop mode, the display unit shows 'S' in the mode field. For the start mode the display unit shows 'r' in the mode field along with temperature and °C and RH in %.

3. **Parameter setting:** To set the temperature in stop mode press set key and required temperature is set by inc and dec keys, press set key to memories value.

4. To set the humidity in stop mode press set key and required RH value is set by inc and dec keys, press set key to memories value.

5. To set the unit timer in stop mode press set key and required time is set by inc and dec keys, press set key to memories value. To run unit without timer set zero in this field.

6. Put sample inside the unit and press start/stop key, display shows 'r' indicating run mode.

7. After set time the unit goes in to stop mode and display indicates 'S'. If time is not set press start/stop key, to manually put unit in stop mode.

Precaution and maintenance
1. Clean the chamber and the shelves at regular intervals.
2. Clean the air cooled condenser at regular intervals which is placed bottom of the machine.
3. Clean the boiler tank and its related accessories periodically.

21. SOP for Homogenizer

Principle: Forced circular movement of the impeller homogenizes the sample.

Operating procedure
1. Switch on the motor.
2. Adjust the shaft height to central half of solution/mixture.
3. Adjust the speed using 'speed' knob.
4. Switch off the motor, after completion of mixing/stirring.
5. Remove the beaker after impeller has stopped (if required).

Precaution and maintenance
1. Clean the shaft before and after use.
2. Calibrate the instrument once a month.

22. SOP for Mass Mixer

Principle: Mixing of wet as well as dry or lump material, especially suited for tablet granulation

Operating procedure
1. Press the "on" key on the display of mass mixer.
2. Set the rpm from the control panel.
3. Speed was regulated with the help of regulator.
4. Start the motor.
5. After the set time, stop the motor and remove the mixture and clean the chamber.
6. Switch off the power supply.

Precaution and maintenance
1. The motor driven machine is also equipped with safety switch to automatically stop the mixer as soon as the cover id opened.
2. After using the mixer clean the paddle and drum properly.

23. SOP for Pfizer Hardness Tester

Principle: A Pfizer hardness tester measures the breaking strength of tablet by applying the principle of pressure and force.

Operating procedure

1. Hold one table t between the two faces provided by pushing forward the movable face by turning the plunger clockwise. Coincide the 'zero' in the scale with the pointer.
2. Enclose front part where tablet is held in sample polybag.
3. Start applying pressure on the tablet by gently rotating the plunger.
4. When the tablet breaks, note the hardness (in kg/sq.cm) directly from the scale.
5. In case, if the pointer is in between the two divisions of scale, read the hardness as 0.5 kg/sq.cm.
6. Discard the broken tablets in water and sample polybag in waste bin.

Precaution and maintenance

1. After use, clean the hardness tester with potable water followed by 0.1% SLS solution followed by potable water to remove the SLS solution and finally rinsed with purified water, and cleans with lint free cloth and keep in its box.
2. This procedure is to be followed during product change over and at the end of shift.

24. SOP for Single Punch Machine

Principle: Single-punch tablet press is designed for pressing tablets from variety of granulated materials. It is drive by motor or hand.

Operating procedure

1. Load the lubricated blend in the hopper for easy setting of thickness and hardness.
2. Set the compression force of machine by force setting wheel.
3. Compression and ejection is actuated by revolution of the wheel drive as the arrow is indicated direction on wheel.
4. After completion of compression of tablets switch off the main power.
5. Kindly wash and clean the machine and its parts.

Precaution and maintenance

1. Before operating the machine ensure that all parts are cleaned. It should be rust and dust free.
2. There should not be any residue of previously used material.
3. Clean the punches and dies with isopropyl alcohol before operating machine.
4. Do not run the machine without any lubricated blend.